Advancements in Athlete Injury Repair: The Role of Mesenchymal Stem Cells

About the Author

Meet Dr. James Utley, PhD. He's not your typical Immunohematology guru. For over two decades, he's been crafting a niche in cellular therapy across the U.S. A proud alum of Johns Hopkins, he took a detour to the Department of Defense, where he reimagined the whole cellular transfusion scene.

But here's where it gets intriguing: James is a Biohacker at heart. He's been on the cutting edge, self-experimenting and pushing the boundaries of CRISPR and genetic engineering like a true avant-garde scientist.

Then there's his stint at Banner Health. Not just any role, mind you. He was the Technical Director of all the blood banks and transfusion services, overseeing a monumental 150K successful cellular transfusions with his artisanal touch. But James isn't just about numbers. He's penned thoughts in some of the most avant-garde medical journals and has been the force behind some truly innovative FDA-approved breakthroughs.

And here's the kicker: this former Navy Scientist traded in his lab coat to chart the unexplored waters of the stem cell revolution. Some even call him the "pirate" of the cellular world. Now, as the Chief Scientific Officer at Auragens, he's making waves and a difference in the world every single day. Cheers to the unconventional trailblazer and world-changer!

www.auragens.com | Instagram: @theauragens | @dr.james.utley

About the Co-Author

With over twenty years of experience as a realistic visionary and a beneficial entrepreneur, Dr. Dan Briggs is the Founder, President, and CEO of multiple successful companies.

In the medical field Dan is the Founder, President & CEO of Auragens, the premier stem cell and research center in the world and located in Panama City, Panama. Spanning the entire 48th floor of the Oceania Business Tower, Auragens has created the world's leading research facility and has attracted top PhD's and medical doctors from the Americas and Europe in its pursuit to improve the standard of care and treatment. He formed a 501c3 nonprofit, primary care company, The Neighborhood Clinic, where he also serves as Chairman and CEO. With multiple locations The Neighborhood Clinic's doctors, and nurse practitioners, can see up to 500 underserved and rural patients per day that previously had no access to medical care. Dan also founded MDX Labs Inc, a CLIA and COLA Certified, high complexity lab network headquartered in Henderson, Nevada. A frontrunner and innovator in the molecular & clinical diagnostics space, MDX was recognized as "Top Small Business" and "Best Workplace" in Nevada. Additionally, and to further his passion in supporting the community Dan founded and serves as Chairman of FOUNDA-TIONS, a 501c3 charitable organization, that provides support and donations to charities globally assisting those in need and breaking down barriers in access to healthcare. In 2023, Dr. Dan Briggs was named Healthcare Executive of the Year by Nevada Business Magazine and a jury of his peers.

Along with his role in his companies, Dan also has served, and continues to serve, on several boards where he acts as advisor, trustee, and mentor. These include NeoVolta (NASDAQ: NEOV), University of Northwestern Ohio (UNOH), Las Vegas HEALS, and Big Brothers Big Sisters.

Dan's career has firm roots in public health, policy, and advocacy, long-held personal passions of his. Dan was a member of the advance team of President George W. Bush during the first US and Russia Summit with Vladimir Putin, held in St. Petersburg, Russia. Dan then oversaw campaigns on behalf of the Governor of California for the Office of Members Services. After relocating to Nevada, Dan was a Founding Member of the Las Vegas World Affairs Council -- a bipartisan organization dedicated to engaging and educating Americans on international affairs and foreign policy. His desire for public service resulted in him being recruited to run as a candidate for the Nevada State Assembly District 20 in 2008. He lost.

Dan earned his Doctorate Degrees in Public Health (DrPH) and Doctor of Laws (LLD) from University of Northwestern Ohio, studied law at Thomas Jefferson School of Law in San Diego, earned his master's degree in Russian, East European, and Eurasian Studies at Stanford University, and an undergraduate degree in Political Science from Pepperdine University. He is married with three children and splits his time between the USA and Panama.

Disclaimer

The content provided in this book is for informational and educational purposes only and is not intended as, nor should it be considered a substitute for, professional medical advice. Do not use the information in this book for diagnosing or treating any medical or health condition. If you have or suspect you have a medical problem, promptly consult your professional healthcare provider. Always seek the advice of your physician or other qualified health provider with any questions you may have regarding a medical condition. Never disregard professional medical advice or delay in seeking it because of something you have read in this book.

Contents

1

Introduction

Background and Significance

In recent years, there has been a growing interest in the regenerative potential of mesenchymal stem cells (MSCs) in the field of athlete injury repair. MSCs are a type of adult stem cell that can be isolated from various sources, including human umbilical cord tissue, specifically Wharton's jelly. These cells have shown promising results in promoting tissue regeneration and facilitating the healing process in athletes with sports-related injuries (Yin et al.).

Athletes are prone to various types of injuries, ranging from muscle strains and ligament tears to bone fractures. These injuries can significantly impact an athlete's performance and career. Traditional treatment approaches, such as surgery and physical therapy, have limitations in terms of efficacy and recovery time. Therefore, there is a need for alternative therapies that can enhance the healing process and promote tissue regeneration (Shukla et al., 2020).

MSCs have gained attention due to their unique characteristics and regenerative properties. These cells have the ability to differentiate into various cell types, including bone, cartilage, and muscle cells. Additionally, MSCs can secrete a wide range of bioactive molecules, such as growth factors, cytokines, and chemokines, which play a crucial role in tissue repair and regeneration (Shukla et al., 2020).

One of the key advantages of using MSCs isolated from human umbilical cord tissue, is their abundant availability. The umbilical cord is a rich source of MSCs, and the collection process is non-invasive and does not pose any ethical concerns. Moreover, MSCs derived from Wharton's jelly have shown superior regenerative potential compared to other sources, such as bone marrow or adipose tissue (Yin et al.).

Exosomes, which are small extracellular vesicles secreted by MSCs, have also emerged as a potential therapeutic tool in athlete injury repair. These exosomes contain a variety of bioactive molecules, including proteins, nucleic acids, and lipids, which can modulate cellular processes and promote tissue regeneration. Exosomes derived from MSCs have been shown to possess anti-inflammatory, immunomodulatory, and pro-regenerative properties (Rao et al., 2019).

The regenerative potential of MSCs and their secreted exosomes can be attributed to their mechanisms of action in injury repair. MSCs can directly differentiate into the specific cell types required for tissue regeneration, such as muscle cells or cartilage cells. Additionally, MSCs can modulate the immune response and reduce inflammation at the injury site, creating a favorable environment for tissue repair. The secreted exosomes can also transfer their cargo of bioactive molecules to recipient cells, promoting cellular proliferation, angiogenesis, and extracellular matrix remodeling (Zhang et al., 2021).

Clinical applications of MSCs and exosome therapies in athlete injury repair have shown promising results. Several studies have reported successful outcomes in the treatment of various sports-related injuries, including tendon and ligament tears, muscle strains, and cartilage defects. MSC-based therapies have demonstrated improved healing rates, reduced pain, and enhanced functional recovery in athletes (Rao et al., 2019).

Despite the potential benefits, there are challenges and limitations associated with the use of MSCs and exosome therapies in athlete injury repair. These include the need for standardized protocols for cell isolation, expansion, and delivery, as well as the potential for immune rejection and tumorigenicity. Additionally, regulatory considerations and safety concerns need to be addressed to ensure the widespread and ethical use of these therapies in athletes (Shukla et al., 2020).

In conclusion, the regenerative potential of MSCs and their secreted exosomes holds great promise in athlete injury repair. MSCs harvested from the Wharton's jelly of human umbilical cord tissue possess distinctive properties that render them the best candidate for therapeutic uses.
Further research and clinical studies are needed to optimize the protocols, address the challenges, and establish the long-term safety and efficacy of MSC-based therapies in athletes (Yin et al.)

Scope and Objectives

The scope of this book is to explore the regenerative potential of mesenchymal stem cells (MSCs) in athlete injury repair, with a specific focus on the therapeutic significance of these cells (Patel, Shah, & Srivastava, 2013). The objectives of this book are to provide insights into the mechanisms of action of MSCs in injury repair, discuss their clinical applications in athletes, and highlight the challenges and limitations associated with their use (Miceli et al., 2021). Additionally, this book aims to examine the role of exosome therapies, which are secreted by MSCs, in regenerative processes and their potential therapeutic applications in athlete injury repair (Hade, Suire, & Suo, 2021).

The use of MSCs in injury repair has gained significant attention in recent years due to their unique regenerative properties. MSCs are multipotent stem cells that can differentiate into various cell types, including osteoblasts, chondrocytes, and adipocytes (Kim, Lee, Xu, Zhang, & Le, 2021). These cells have the ability to self-renew and possess immunomodulatory properties, making them an attractive option for regenerative medicine (Patel, Shah, & Srivastava, 2013).

The first objective of this book is to provide a comprehensive understanding of the characteristics of MSCs. MSCs can be isolated from various sources, including bone marrow, adipose tissue, and umbilical cord tissue. However, this book will specifically focus on MSCs isolated from human umbilical cord tissue, specifically Wharton's jelly (Miceli et al., 2021). Wharton's jelly is a gelatinous substance found in the umbilical cord that contains a rich source of MSCs. These MSCs have been shown to have superior regenerative potential compared to MSCs derived from other sources (Patel, Shah, & Srivastava, 2013).

The second objective is to explore the mechanisms of action of MSCs in injury repair. MSCs have been found to exert their regenerative effects through various mechanisms, including differentiation into specific cell types, secretion of growth factors and cytokines, and modulation of the immune response (Kim, Lee, Xu, Zhang, & Le, 2021). These mechanisms play a crucial role in promoting tissue regeneration and reducing inflammation, thereby facilitating the healing process in athletes (Hade, Suire, & Suo, 2021).

The third objective is to discuss the clinical applications of MSCs in athlete injury repair. Numerous studies have demonstrated the efficacy of MSC-based therapies in treating various sports-related injuries, such as ligament tears, muscle strains, and cartilage damage (Miceli et al., 2021). This book will provide an overview of the different approaches used in MSC-based therapies, including direct injection of MSCs into the injured site, as well as the use of MSC-derived exosomes (Hade, Suire, & Suo, 2021).

The fourth objective is to address the challenges and limitations associated with the use of MSCs in athlete injury repair. Despite their promising regenerative potential, there are several factors that need to be considered when utilizing MSCs in a clinical setting. These include the optimal dosage and timing of MSC administration, the potential for immune rejection, and the need for standardized protocols for MSC isolation and expansion (Kim, Lee, Xu, Zhang, & Le, 2021). By addressing these challenges, this book aims to provide a comprehensive understanding of the current limitations and future directions for MSC-based therapies in athletes (Patel, Shah, & Srivastava, 2013).

In addition to MSCs, this book will also explore the role of exosome therapies in athlete injury repair. Exosomes are small extracellular vesicles secreted by MSCs that contain a variety of bioactive molecules, including proteins, nucleic acids, and growth factors (Hade, Suire, & Suo, 2021). These exosomes have been shown to possess regenerative properties and can modulate various cellular processes involved in tissue repair (Miceli et al., 2021). The therapeutic applications of exosomes in athlete injury repair will be discussed, along with the safety and regulatory considerations associated with their use (Kim, Lee, Xu, Zhang, & Le, 2021).

Overall, the scope of this book is to provide a comprehensive overview of the regenerative potential of MSCs and exosome therapies in athlete injury repair. By examining the mechanisms of action, clinical applications, challenges, and limitations of these therapies, this book aims to contribute to the growing body of knowledge in the field of regenerative medicine and provide insights for future research and clinical practice (Patel, Shah, & Srivastava, 2013).

Selection of Mesenchymal Stem Cells

Wharton's jelly is a gelatinous substance found within the umbilical cord, which contains a rich source of MSCs. These MSCs have been shown to possess unique regenerative properties and a higher proliferation capacity compared to other sources of MSCs, such as bone marrow or adipose tissue (Abouelnaga et al., 2022; Çiçek & Bağcı, 2023).

The decision to focus on MSCs derived from Wharton's jelly was also influenced by the ethical considerations associated with their collection. The use of umbilical cord tissue for MSC isolation does not involve any invasive procedures or harm to the donor, making it an ethically favorable source of MSCs for research purposes (Radhakrishnan et al., 2021; Gallicchio, 2023).

Overview of Mesenchymal Stem Cells and Exosome Therapies

Mesenchymal stem cells (MSCs) have gained significant attention in the field of regenerative medicine due to their unique regenerative properties. These cells have the ability to differentiate into various cell types and possess immunomodulatory and anti-inflammatory properties (Kim et al., 2021). In addition to their direct regenerative potential, MSCs also secrete extracellular vesicles called exosomes, which play a crucial role in intercellular communication and tissue repair (Jagiełło et al., 2019). This section provides an overview of MSCs and exosome therapies, focusing specifically on those isolated from human umbilical cord tissue. (Sriramulu et al., 2018; Sadlik et al., 2017).

Characteristics of Mesenchymal Stem Cells

MSCs possess several unique characteristics that make them ideal for regenerative therapies. Firstly, they have the ability to self-renew, meaning they can divide and produce more MSCs. This property ensures a sustainable source of cells for therapeutic applications. Secondly, MSCs have the potential to differentiate into multiple cell types, including bone, cartilage, muscle, and fat cells (Okić-Đorđević et al., 2021). This multilineage differentiation capacity allows them to contribute to tissue repair and regeneration.

Furthermore, MSCs exhibit immunomodulatory properties, which means they can regulate the immune response and reduce inflammation (Che et al., 2022). This ability makes them particularly valuable in the context of athlete injury repair, as inflammation is a common response to tissue damage. By modulating the immune response, MSCs can help create an environment conducive to tissue healing and regeneration (Lim et al., 2021).

Clinical Applications in Athlete Injury Repair

The regenerative potential of MSCs has been extensively studied in the context of athlete injury repair. Various preclinical and clinical studies have demonstrated the efficacy of MSC-based therapies in promoting tissue healing and functional recovery (Berebichez-Fridman et al., 2017). In the field of orthopedics, MSCs have shown promising results in the treatment of conditions such as ligament and tendon injuries, osteoarthritis, and cartilage defects (Shah, 2019). For example, in a clinical trial involving athletes with chronic Achilles tendonitis, MSC injections resulted in improved pain relief and functional outcomes compared to conventional treatments.

MSCs have also been investigated for their potential in treating muscle injuries, such as strains and tears. In a study involving professional soccer players with muscle injuries, MSC injections led to faster recovery and return to play compared to standard rehabilitation protocols (Khan et al., 2012).The regenerative potential of MSCs has been extensively studied in the context of athlete injury repair. Various preclinical and clinical studies have demonstrated the efficacy of MSC-based therapies in promoting tissue healing and functional recovery (Berebichez-Fridman et al., 2017). For example, in a clinical trial involving athletes with chronic Achilles tendonitis, MSC injections resulted in improved pain relief and functional outcomes compared to conventional treatments.

Exosome Therapies in Athlete Injury Repair

Exosomes are small extracellular vesicles secreted by MSCs that play a crucial role in intercellular communication. These vesicles contain a variety of bioactive molecules, including proteins, nucleic acids, and lipids, which can modulate cellular processes and promote tissue repair (Keshtkar, Azarpira, & Ghahremani, 2018).

Exosome therapies have emerged as a promising approach in regenerative medicine, including athlete injury repair. The therapeutic potential of MSC-derived exosomes lies in their ability to transfer bioactive molecules to target cells and modulate their behavior. These molecules can promote cell proliferation, angiogenesis, and tissue regeneration (Bjørge, Kim, Mano, Kalionis, & Chrzanowski, n.d.).

Several studies have demonstrated the efficacy of MSC-derived exosomes in promoting tissue repair in various injury models. For example, in a study on a rat model of muscle injury, treatment with MSC-derived exosomes resulted in enhanced muscle regeneration and functional recovery (Moghadasi et al., 2021). Similarly, in a study on a rabbit model of cartilage injury, exosome therapy promoted cartilage repair and improved joint function (Zhao, Sun, Liu, Ding, She, Mao, Xu, Qian, & Yan, 2019).

Safety and Regulatory Considerations

When considering the clinical application of MSCs and exosome therapies, safety and regulatory considerations are of utmost importance. It is crucial to ensure that these therapies are safe and do not pose any significant risks to the patients.

MSCs derived from human umbilical cord tissue, specifically Wharton's jelly, have shown a favorable safety profile in clinical trials. These cells have low immunogenicity, meaning they are less likely to trigger an immune response when transplanted into a recipient (Negi & Griffin, 2020). Additionally, MSCs have demonstrated a low risk of tumorigenicity, further supporting their safety for therapeutic use (Negi & Griffin, 2020).

Exosome therapies also hold promise in terms of safety. As the therapeutic cargo is contained within the exosomes, the risk of adverse effects associated with direct cell transplantation is minimized (Yin, Wang, & Zhao, 2019). However, further research is needed to fully understand the long-term safety and potential side effects of exosome therapies (Yin, Wang, & Zhao, 2019).

Regulatory agencies play a crucial role in ensuring the safety and efficacy of MSC-based therapies. Strict regulations and guidelines are in place to govern the development and clinical translation of these therapies. Compliance with these regulations is essential to ensure the ethical and responsible use of MSCs and exosome therapies in athlete injury repair (Börger et al., n.d.; Yamatani et al., 2022).

Future Perspectives and Challenges

The field of MSC-based therapies and exosome therapies is rapidly evolving, with ongoing research aimed at further understanding their regenerative potential and optimizing their clinical applications (Ebrahimi et al., 2023). Future studies will likely focus on elucidating the specific mechanisms of action of MSCs and exosomes, identifying optimal dosing and delivery methods, and exploring their potential in combination with other regenerative strategies (Zeng, 2023).

Despite the promising results, several challenges need to be addressed to fully harness the regenerative potential of MSCs and exosome therapies. These challenges include standardization of isolation and characterization methods, optimization of manufacturing processes, and addressing the variability in therapeutic outcomes observed in different patient populations (Kosanović et al., 2023).

In conclusion, Mesenchymal stem cells sourced from the Wharton's jelly of human umbilical cord tissue show significant potential for the repair of athletic injuries. Their regenerative properties, including their ability to differentiate into multiple cell types and secrete bioactive molecules, make them an attractive therapeutic option. Furthermore, exosome therapies derived from MSCs offer a novel approach to promote tissue repair and regeneration. However, further research and clinical trials are needed to fully understand the mechanisms of action, optimize therapeutic protocols, and ensure the safety and efficacy of these regenerative therapies (Labusek et al., 2023).

2

Regenerative Treatment Strategies for Athletic Injury Recovery

Mesenchymal Stem Cells possess unique regenerative properties that make them an ideal candidate for therapeutic applications in sports medicine (Miceli et al., 2021). In addition to their inherent regenerative potential, MSCs also secrete exosomes, which further enhance their therapeutic effects (Hade et al., 2021). This section will explore the therapeutic applications of MSCs and exosome therapies in athlete injury repair, focusing on their regenerative potential and the mechanisms underlying their therapeutic significance.

Regenerative Potential of MSCs in Athlete Injury Repair

MSCs have gained significant attention in the field of regenerative medicine due to their ability to differentiate into various cell types and their immunomodulatory properties (Margiana et al., 2022). When it comes to athlete injury repair, MSCs have shown promising results in promoting tissue regeneration and accelerating the healing process.

One of the key regenerative properties of MSCs is their ability to differentiate into different cell lineages, including osteoblasts, chondrocytes, and myocytes. This differentiation potential allows MSCs to contribute to the repair and regeneration of injured tissues, such as bones, cartilage, and muscles (Miceli et al., 2021). By differentiating into the specific cell types required for tissue repair, MSCs can aid in the restoration of the injured tissue's structure and function.

Furthermore, MSCs secrete various growth factors, cytokines, and chemokines that promote tissue regeneration and modulate the inflammatory response. These paracrine factors have been shown to stimulate angiogenesis, enhance cell proliferation, and promote extracellular matrix synthesis (Ghafouri-Fard et al., 2021). By creating a favorable microenvironment for tissue repair, MSCs can facilitate the healing process and improve the outcomes of athlete injury repair.

Exosome Therapies in Athlete Injury Repair

Exosomes are small extracellular vesicles secreted by MSCs that play a crucial role in intercellular communication. These vesicles contain a diverse range of bioactive molecules, including proteins, nucleic acids, and lipids, which can be transferred to recipient cells and modulate their function (Hade et al., 2021). In the context of athlete injury repair, exosomes derived from MSCs have shown immense therapeutic potential.

Exosomes secreted by MSCs have been found to possess similar regenerative properties as their parent cells. They can promote tissue regeneration, modulate the inflammatory response, and enhance the healing process (Hade et al., 2021). The bioactive molecules encapsulated within exosomes, such as growth factors, microRNAs, and cytokines, can regulate various cellular processes involved in tissue repair (Ghafouri-Fard et al., 2021).

One of the key advantages of exosome therapies is their ability to bypass the limitations associated with cell-based therapies. Exosomes can be easily isolated, purified, and stored, making them a more practical and scalable option for therapeutic applications (Ghafouri-Fard et al., 2021). Additionally, exosomes derived from MSCs have shown excellent stability and can be delivered to the injured site via various routes, including intravenous injection, local administration, and tissue engineering scaffolds (Hade et al., 2021).

Mechanisms of Action in Athlete Injury Repair

Both MSCs and exosomes exert their therapeutic effects through multiple mechanisms, which contribute to their regenerative potential in athlete injury repair. These mechanisms include:

1. **Immunomodulation:** MSCs and exosomes can modulate the immune response by suppressing pro-inflammatory cytokines and promoting anti-inflammatory factors (Margiana et al., 2022). This immunomodulatory effect helps to reduce

inflammation at the site of injury and create a favorable environment for tissue repair.

2. **Angiogenesis:** MSCs and exosomes promote the formation of new blood vessels, a process known as angiogenesis (Miceli et al., 2021). This is crucial for supplying oxygen and nutrients to the injured tissue, facilitating its regeneration and repair.

3. **Cellular Differentiation:** MSCs have the ability to differentiate into various cell types, including osteoblasts, chondrocytes, and myocytes (Miceli et al., 2021). This differentiation potential allows MSCs to directly contribute to tissue regeneration and repair.

4. **Extracellular Matrix Remodeling:** MSCs and exosomes can stimulate the synthesis and remodeling of the extracellular matrix, which is essential for tissue regeneration. They promote the deposition of collagen and other matrix components, enhancing the structural integrity of the repaired tissue (Ghafouri-Fard et al., 2021).

5. **Paracrine Signaling:** MSCs and exosomes secrete a wide range of bioactive molecules, including growth factors, cytokines, and microRNAs. These molecules can modulate various cellular processes involved in tissue repair, such as cell proliferation, migration, and differentiation (Hade et al., 2021).

By harnessing these mechanisms, MSCs and exosomes hold great potential for promoting athlete injury repair and improving the outcomes of regenerative therapies.

Clinical Applications and Future Perspectives

The therapeutic applications of MSCs and exosome therapies in athlete injury repair are still in the early stages of clinical translation. However, several preclinical and clinical studies have shown promising results, demonstrating the safety and efficacy of these regenerative approaches (Margiana et al., 2022)

3

Regenerative Potential of Mesenchymal Stem Cells (MSC)

Properties of Mesenchymal Stem Cells

Mesenchymal stem cells (MSCs) are a type of adult stem cell that hold great promise in the field of regenerative medicine. These cells have the ability to differentiate into various cell types, including bone, cartilage, muscle, and fat cells (Samsonraj et al., 2017). MSCs are characterized by their self-renewal capacity (Fu et al., 2019) and their ability to migrate to sites of injury or inflammation (Miana &

González, 2018), making them an attractive option for the repair and regeneration of damaged tissues in athletes. The extracellular vesicles derived from MSCs, particularly exosomes, have also been identified as a key factor in mediating these regenerative processes (Taghdiri Nooshabadi et al., 2018).

Source of Mesenchymal Stem Cells

The choice to use MSCs derived from the Wharton's jelly of human umbilical cord tissue was influenced by a variety of considerations. Wharton's jelly is a gelatinous substance found within the umbilical cord, which contains a rich source of MSCs. These MSCs have been shown to possess unique regenerative properties and a higher proliferation capacity compared to other sources of MSCs, such as bone marrow or adipose tissue (Negargar et al., 2022). The decision to focus on MSCs derived from Wharton's jelly was also influenced by the ethical considerations associated with their collection. The use of umbilical cord tissue for MSC isolation does not involve any invasive procedures or harm to the donor, making it an ethically favorable source of MSCs for research purposes (Lelek & Zuba-Surma, 2020).

Immunophenotype of Mesenchymal Stem Cells

One of the defining characteristics of MSCs is their immunophenotype. MSCs are typically positive for specific surface markers, such as CD73, CD90, and CD105, while being negative for markers such as CD45 and CD34 (Usupzhanova et al., 2023; Heyman et al., 2023). This immunophenotype allows for the identification and isolation of MSCs from other cell types present in the umbilical cord tissue.

Multipotency and Differentiation Potential

MSCs are multipotent cells, meaning they have the ability to differentiate into multiple cell lineages (Salimi et al., 2021). Under appropriate conditions, MSCs can differentiate into osteoblasts (bone cells), chondrocytes (cartilage cells), adipocytes (fat cells), and myocytes (muscle cells) (Mathieu & Loboa, 2012). This multipotency makes MSCs a valuable tool for tissue regeneration and repair in athletes with various types of injuries (Kangari et al., 2020; Li et al., 2021).

Paracrine Signaling and Trophic Effects

Mesenchymal Stem Cells (MSCs) manifest regenerative capabilities via paracrine mechanisms and trophic influences. MSCs are prolific in the secretion of an array of bioactive molecules encompassing growth factors, cytokines, and chemokines. These molecules are instrumental in the modulation of the local cellular milieu, thereby facilitating tissue regeneration (Tamama & Kerpedjieva, 2012). Empirical evidence has demonstrated that these secreted factors induce angiogenesis, attenuate inflammatory responses, and enhance cellular viability and proliferation (Cavaliere, Donno, & D'Ambrosi, 2015; Quaglia et al., 2020). Furthermore, the paracrine action of MSCs has been implicated in modulating cell death, thereby contributing to the restoration of cellular function and organ homeostasis (Naji et al., 2019).

Immunomodulatory Properties

MSCs possess unique immunomodulatory properties that make them particularly suitable for the treatment of athlete injuries. These cells have the ability to suppress the immune response and modulate the activity of various immune cells, such as T cells, B cells, and natural killer cells (Miguel et al., 2012; Zhang et al., 2010). By suppressing excessive inflammation and promoting a balanced immune response, MSCs can create an optimal environment for tissue repair and regeneration (Rafieerad et al., 2019; McTaggart & Atkinson, 2007).

Low Immunogenicity

One of the advantages of using MSCs for regenerative purposes is their low immunogenicity. MSCs express low levels of major histocompatibility complex (MHC) class II molecules and co-stimulatory molecules, making them less likely to be recognized and attacked by the recipient's immune system (Inoue et al., 2006). This low immunogenicity reduces the risk of immune rejection and allows for the use of allogeneic MSCs from unrelated donors (Avivar-Valderas et al., 2019; Nishizawa & Seki, 2016).

Proliferative Capacity and Expansion Potential

MSCs have a high proliferative capacity, allowing for their expansion in culture without losing their regenerative properties (Mushahary et al., 2018). This ability to expand MSCs in large quantities is crucial for their clinical application, as it ensures an adequate supply of cells for therapeutic purposes (Kim & Park, 2017). However, it is important to note that the expansion process should be carefully controlled to maintain the quality and functionality of the MSCs (Yang et al., 2018; Li et al., 2015).

Safety Considerations

When considering the use of MSCs for athlete injury repair, safety is of utmost importance. Extensive preclinical and clinical studies have been conducted to evaluate the safety profile of MSCs. These studies have shown that MSCs are generally safe and well-tolerated, with minimal adverse effects reported (Deans & Moseley, 2000; Smith et al., 2013). However, it is essential to adhere to strict quality control measures and follow regulatory guidelines to ensure the safety and efficacy of MSC-based therapies (Hoogduijn & Dor, 2011).

In conclusion, MSCs isolated from human umbilical cord tissue, specifically Wharton's jelly, possess unique characteristics and regenerative properties that make them an ideal candidate for athlete injury repair. These cells exhibit multipotency, immunomodulatory properties, and the ability to secrete bioactive molecules that promote tissue repair and regeneration (Imberti et al., 2011; Menge et al., 2012). Furthermore, their low immunogenicity and safety profile make them a promising option for allogeneic transplantation (Kramer et al., 2012). However, further research and clinical studies are needed to fully understand the mechanisms of action and optimize the therapeutic potential of MSCs in athlete injury repair (Oliveira et al., 2019).

4

MSC: Mechanisms of Action in Injury Repair

Mechanisms of Action in Injury Repair (MSC)

Mesenchymal stem cells (MSCs) derived from human umbilical cord tissue, specifically Wharton's jelly, have shown immense potential in the field of injury repair in athletes. These cells possess unique regenerative properties that enable them to promote tissue healing and regeneration (Caplan, 1991). In addition to their direct therapeutic effects, MSCs also secrete exosomes, which play a crucial role in mediating the regenerative processes (Lai et al., 2011).

Paracrine Signaling in Injury Repair (MSC)

One of the primary mechanisms through which MSCs exert their regenerative effects is paracrine signaling. MSCs have the ability to secrete a wide range of bioactive molecules, including growth factors, cytokines, and chemokines. These molecules act as signaling molecules that can modulate the local microenvironment and promote tissue repair (Caplan & Correa, 2011). For example, MSCs release factors such as vascular endothelial growth factor (VEGF), fibroblast growth factor (FGF), and transforming growth factor-beta (TGF-β), which stimulate angiogenesis, promote cell proliferation, and enhance tissue remodeling (Caplan & Correa, 2011).

The paracrine signaling of MSCs is not limited to the injured site but can also affect neighboring cells and tissues. This ability allows MSCs to exert their regenerative effects beyond their immediate vicinity, making them a promising therapeutic option for widespread injuries or conditions.

Immunomodulation in Injury Repair (MSC)

In addition to their paracrine signaling, MSCs possess potent immunomodulatory properties. They can modulate the immune response by suppressing the activation and proliferation of immune cells, such as T cells, B cells, and natural killer cells (Bartholomew et al., 2002). MSCs also promote the generation of regulatory T cells (Tregs) and shift the immune response towards an anti-inflammatory phenotype (Bartholomew et al., 2002).

By modulating the immune response, MSCs create an environment that is conducive to tissue repair. Inflammation is a crucial component of the healing process, but excessive or prolonged inflammation can impede proper tissue regeneration. MSCs help regulate the inflammatory response, preventing excessive inflammation and promoting a balanced immune environment that supports tissue repair.

Differentiation and Regeneration in Injury Repair (MSC)

MSCs have the ability to differentiate into various cell types, including osteoblasts, chondrocytes, and adipocytes. This multilineage differentiation potential allows MSCs to contribute directly to tissue regeneration by replacing damaged or lost cells (Pittenger et al., 1999). In the context of athlete injury repair, MSCs can differentiate into specific cell types found in musculoskeletal tissues, such as cartilage, bone, and muscle cells.

Furthermore, MSCs can stimulate the proliferation and differentiation of endogenous stem cells present in the injured tissue. This paracrine effect enhances the regenerative capacity of the injured tissue by promoting the recruitment and activation of local stem cells (Pittenger et al., 1999).

Clinical Applications in Athlete Injury Repair (MSC)

Mesenchymal stem cells (MSCs) derived from human umbilical cord tissue, specifically Wharton's jelly, have shown great promise in the field of athlete injury repair. These cells possess unique regenerative properties that make them an ideal candidate for treating various types of sports-related injuries. In this section, we will explore the clinical applications of MSCs in athlete injury repair and discuss their therapeutic significance.

Ligament and Tendon Injuries

Ligament and tendon injuries are common among athletes and can significantly impact their performance and overall well-being. Traditional treatment options for these injuries often involve surgical intervention, which may have limitations and lengthy recovery periods. However, MSC-based therapies have emerged as a promising alternative for promoting tissue regeneration and accelerating the healing process.

Studies have shown that MSCs have the ability to differentiate into tenocytes, the cells responsible for tendon formation and repair. When injected into the injured area, MSCs can promote the production of collagen and other extracellular matrix components, leading to enhanced tissue healing and improved biomechanical properties of the injured ligament or tendon. Furthermore, MSCs have been found to possess immunomodulatory properties, reducing inflammation and preventing excessive scar tissue formation (Caplan, 1991; Bartholomew et al., 2002).

Cartilage Repair

Articular cartilage injuries, such as those occurring in the knee joint, are a common concern for athletes. These injuries often result from repetitive trauma or overuse, leading to pain, joint dysfunction, and the development of osteoarthritis. MSCs have shown great potential in promoting cartilage repair and regeneration, making them a valuable tool in the treatment of these injuries.

When MSCs are introduced into the damaged cartilage, they can differentiate into chondrocytes, the cells responsible for cartilage formation (Pittenger et al., 1999). This differentiation process is facilitated by the presence of specific growth factors and signaling molecules in the joint microenvironment. MSCs also secrete various bioactive factors that promote the proliferation and differentiation of endogenous chondrocytes, further enhancing the regenerative process (Caplan & Correa, 2011).

Clinical studies have demonstrated the efficacy of MSC-based therapies in improving cartilage repair and reducing pain in athletes with cartilage injuries. These therapies have the potential to delay or even prevent the progression of osteoarthritis, providing athletes with a better chance of returning to their sport at full capacity.

Muscle Injuries

Muscle injuries, such as strains and tears, are common in athletes, particularly those involved in high-impact sports. These injuries can significantly impact an athlete's performance and require a comprehensive and efficient treatment approach. MSCs have shown promise in promoting muscle regeneration and accelerating the healing process in these injuries.

When MSCs are injected into the injured muscle, they can differentiate into myocytes, the cells responsible for muscle formation and repair. This differentiation process is facilitated by the presence of specific growth factors and signaling molecules in the injured muscle microenvironment. MSCs also secrete various factors that promote angiogenesis, the formation of new blood vessels, which is crucial for delivering oxygen and nutrients to the regenerating muscle tissue (Caplan, 1991; Caplan & Correa, 2011).

Clinical studies have demonstrated the potential of MSC-based therapies in improving muscle regeneration and functional recovery in athletes with muscle injuries. These therapies have shown promising results in reducing pain, promoting tissue healing, and restoring muscle strength and function.

Bone Fractures

Bone fractures are common in athletes, particularly those involved in contact sports or activities with repetitive impact. Traditional treatment options for bone fractures often involve immobilization and surgical intervention, which may have limitations and lengthy recovery periods. MSC-based therapies have emerged as a potential alternative for promoting bone healing and accelerating the recovery process.

When MSCs are introduced into the site of the fracture, they can differentiate into osteoblasts, the cells responsible for bone formation and repair (Pittenger et al., 1999). MSCs also secrete various factors that promote angiogenesis and the recruitment of other cells involved in bone healing, such as osteoclasts and mesenchymal progenitor cells. This coordinated response leads to enhanced bone regeneration and accelerated fracture healing (Caplan & Correa, 2011).

Clinical studies have shown promising results in the use of MSC-based therapies for promoting bone healing in athletes with fractures. These therapies have the potential to reduce the recovery time, improve bone union, and enhance the overall functional outcome.

Neurological Injuries

Neurological injuries, such as traumatic brain injuries and spinal cord injuries, can have devastating consequences for athletes. These injuries often result in long-term disabilities and may require lifelong care. MSC-based therapies have shown promise in promoting neurological recovery and functional restoration in these injuries.

When MSCs are introduced into the injured area, they can secrete various factors that promote neuroprotection, reduce inflammation, and enhance tissue repair. MSCs also have the ability to differentiate into neural-like cells and integrate into the damaged neural tissue, providing structural support and promoting functional recovery (Caplan, 1991; Bartholomew et al., 2002).

Clinical studies have demonstrated the potential of MSC-based therapies in improving neurological outcomes in athletes with traumatic brain injuries and spinal cord injuries. These therapies have shown promising results in reducing inflammation, promoting tissue repair, and enhancing functional recovery.

In conclusion, MSC-based therapies derived from human umbilical cord tissue, specifically Wharton's jelly, have shown great potential in the clinical applications of athlete injury repair. These therapies have demonstrated their regenerative properties in promoting ligament and tendon repair, cartilage regeneration, muscle healing, bone fracture healing, and neurological recovery. Further research and clinical trials are needed to optimize the protocols and ensure the long-term safety and efficacy of these therapies.

Extracellular Vesicles and Exosome Therapies

Apart from their direct regenerative effects, MSCs secrete extracellular vesicles, including exosomes, which play a crucial role in mediating the therapeutic benefits of MSC-based therapies. Exosomes are small membrane-bound vesicles that contain various bioactive molecules, including proteins, nucleic acids, and lipids. These exosomes can be taken up by recipient cells, where they deliver their cargo and modulate cellular functions (Lai et al., 2011).

Exosomes derived from MSCs have been shown to possess similar regenerative properties as their parent cells. They can promote angiogenesis, reduce inflammation, and enhance tissue repair. The cargo of exosomes includes growth factors, microRNAs, and other signaling molecules that can regulate cellular processes involved in injury repair. This will be covered in depth in the next chapter.

5

Exosome Therapies in Athlete Injury Repair (MSC-Exos)

Exosomes are small extracellular vesicles that are secreted by various cell types, including mesenchymal stem cells (MSCs). These vesicles play a crucial role in intercellular communication and have emerged as promising therapeutic agents in regenerative medicine (Yuan et al., 2023). In this section, we will explore the biogenesis and composition of exosomes, focusing specifically on those derived from human umbilical cord tissue and Wharton's jelly-derived MSCs.

Biogenesis of Exosomes

Exosomes are formed through a complex process involving the endosomal pathway. It begins with the invagination of the plasma membrane, resulting in the formation of early endosomes. These early endosomes then mature into late endosomes, also known as multivesicular bodies (MVBs). Within the MVBs, intraluminal vesicles (ILVs) are generated through the inward budding of the endosomal membrane. These ILVs are subsequently released into the extracellular space upon fusion of the MVBs with the plasma membrane, giving rise to exosomes (Hade et al., 2021).

The biogenesis of exosomes is tightly regulated and involves various molecular machinery, including the endosomal sorting complex required for transport (ESCRT) machinery. The ESCRT machinery consists of several protein complexes (ESCRT-0, -I, -II, and -III) that facilitate the sorting of specific cargo molecules into ILVs. Additionally, other proteins, such as Alix and tetraspanins (e.g., CD9, CD63, and CD81), are involved in the formation and release of exosomes (Savary et al., 2023).

Composition of Exosomes

Exosomes are composed of a lipid bilayer membrane that encapsulates a diverse array of bioactive molecules, including proteins, lipids, nucleic acids, and various signaling molecules. The cargo carried by exosomes is highly dependent on the cell type of origin and the physiological or pathological conditions of the cell (Janockova et al., 2021).

Proteomic analysis of exosomes derived from human umbilical cord tissue and Wharton's jelly-derived MSCs has revealed the presence of numerous proteins involved in cell adhesion, immune modulation, tissue repair, and angiogenesis. These proteins include integrins, growth factors (such as vascular endothelial growth factor and fibroblast growth factor), cytokines, chemokines, and extracellular matrix components. The presence of these proteins suggests that exosomes derived from MSCs have the potential to modulate various cellular processes involved in tissue regeneration and repair (Yuan et al., 2023).

In addition to proteins, exosomes also contain various types of nucleic acids, including messenger RNA (mRNA), microRNA (miRNA), and long non-coding RNA (lncRNA). These nucleic acids can be transferred to recipient cells upon uptake of exosomes, thereby influencing gene expression and cellular functions. The transfer of functional RNA molecules through exosomes has been shown to regulate processes such as cell proliferation, differentiation, and immune modulation (Hade et al., 2021).

Furthermore, exosomes derived from MSCs have been found to contain lipids, including cholesterol, sphingomyelin, and phospholipids. These lipids not only contribute to the structural integrity of exosomes but also play a role in their biological functions. For example, certain lipids present in exosomes have been shown to modulate immune responses and promote tissue regeneration (Savary et al., 2023).

Cargo Sorting and Selective Packaging

The selective packaging of cargo molecules into exosomes is a highly regulated process that involves specific sorting mechanisms. The sorting of cargo molecules into exosomes can occur through both ESCRT-dependent and ESCRT-independent pathways (Janockova et al., 2021).

The ESCRT-dependent pathway involves the recognition of specific protein motifs, such as ubiquitin, by the ESCRT machinery. This recognition leads to the sequestration of cargo molecules into ILVs, which are subsequently released as exosomes. On the other hand, the ESCRT-independent pathway relies on the interaction of cargo molecules with lipid rafts or tetraspanin-enriched microdomains, leading to their incorporation into exosomes (Yuan et al., 2023).

The cargo sorting process is influenced by various factors, including the cellular environment, cellular stress, and the activation of specific signaling pathways. These factors can modulate the composition of exosomes and their therapeutic potential (Hade et al., 2021).

Heterogeneity of Exosomes

It is important to note that exosomes derived from different cell sources or under different conditions can exhibit heterogeneity in terms of their size, cargo composition, and functional properties. This heterogeneity reflects the dynamic nature of exosomes and highlights the need for standardized isolation and characterization methods (Savary et al., 2023).

To ensure the reproducibility and reliability of exosome-based therapies, it is crucial to establish standardized protocols for the isolation, purification, and characterization of exosomes. This will enable researchers and clinicians to accurately assess the therapeutic potential of exosomes and facilitate their translation into clinical practice (Janockova et al., 2021).

In summary, exosomes derived from human umbilical cord tissue and Wharton's jelly-derived MSCs are small extracellular vesicles that play a vital role in intercellular communication and regenerative processes. These exosomes are composed of a lipid bilayer membrane and carry a diverse cargo of proteins, nucleic acids, lipids, and signaling molecules. The selective packaging of cargo molecules into exosomes is a highly regulated process that involves specific sorting mechanisms. However, the heterogeneity of exosomes derived from different cell sources or under different conditions highlights the need for standardized isolation and characterization methods (Yuan et al., 2023).

Role of Exosomes in Regenerative Processes

Exosomes are small extracellular vesicles that are secreted by various cell types, including mesenchymal stem cells (MSCs). These tiny vesicles play a crucial role in intercellular communication and have emerged as promising therapeutic agents in regenerative medicine (Koga et al., 2023). In recent years, there has been growing interest in understanding the role of exosomes in regenerative processes, particularly in the context of athlete injury repair.

Exosome-Mediated Cell-to-Cell Communication

Exosomes are involved in cell-to-cell communication by transferring bioactive molecules, such as proteins, lipids, and nucleic acids, from donor cells to recipient cells. This transfer of molecular cargo allows exosomes to modulate various cellular processes, including proliferation, differentiation, and immune response (Wang et al., 2023). In the context of athlete injury repair, exosomes derived from MSCs have been shown to promote tissue regeneration and accelerate the healing process.

Exosomes as Carriers of Regenerative Factors

One of the key mechanisms by which exosomes contribute to regenerative processes is through the transfer of regenerative factors. MSC-derived exosomes are enriched with a variety of growth factors, cytokines, and miRNAs that have been shown to promote tissue repair and regeneration (Sun et al., 2021). These regenerative factors can stimulate the proliferation and migration of resident cells at the site of injury, enhance angiogenesis, and modulate the immune response, ultimately leading to tissue regeneration.

1. **Immunomodulatory Effects of Exosomes**

   In addition to their role in delivering regenerative factors, exosomes derived from MSCs also possess potent immunomodulatory properties. These exosomes can modulate the activity of immune cells, such as T cells, B cells, and macrophages, by suppressing pro-inflammatory responses and promoting anti-inflammatory and immunosuppressive pathways (Bellei et al., 2022). By regulating the immune response, exosomes can create a favorable environment for tissue repair and regeneration, particularly in the context of athlete injuries where inflammation can hinder the healing process.

2. **Exosomes and Extracellular Matrix Remodeling**

   Extracellular matrix (ECM) remodeling is a critical process in tissue repair and regeneration. Exosomes derived from MSCs have been shown to play a role in ECM remodeling by regulating the activity of matrix metalloproteinases (MMPs) and tissue inhibitors of metalloproteinases (TIMPs) (Sun et al., 2021). These exosomes can modulate the balance between MMPs and TIMPs, thereby promoting the degradation of damaged ECM components and facilitating the synthesis of new ECM components. This remodeling process is essential for the restoration of tissue structure and function.

3. **Exosomes and Angiogenesis**

Angiogenesis, the formation of new blood vessels, is a crucial process in tissue repair and regeneration. Exosomes derived from MSCs have been shown to promote angiogenesis by stimulating the proliferation, migration, and tube formation of endothelial cells (Sun et al., 2021). These exosomes can deliver pro-angiogenic factors, such as vascular endothelial growth factor (VEGF) and fibroblast growth factor (FGF), to the site of injury, thereby enhancing the formation of new blood vessels and improving blood supply to the damaged tissue.

4. **Exosomes and Anti-Fibrotic Effects**

Fibrosis, the excessive deposition of scar tissue, is a common complication in tissue repair. Exosomes derived from MSCs have been shown to possess anti-fibrotic effects by inhibiting the activation and proliferation of fibroblasts, the cells responsible for scar tissue formation (Bellei et al., 2022). These exosomes can deliver anti-fibrotic factors, such as miRNAs and growth factors, to the site of injury, thereby preventing excessive scar tissue formation and promoting the regeneration of functional tissue.

5. **Synergistic Effects of Exosomes and Mesenchymal Stem Cells**

It is important to note that the regenerative effects of exosomes are not solely attributed to their cargo of bioactive molecules. The interaction between exosomes and MSCs is a complex and dynamic process that involves the exchange of signals and the activation of various signaling pathways. Studies have shown that the co-administration of exosomes and MSCs can enhance the therapeutic efficacy compared to the administration of exosomes or MSCs alone (Koga et al., 2023). This synergistic effect is believed to be due to the complementary actions of exosomes and MSCs in promoting tissue repair and regeneration.

In conclusion, exosomes derived from MSCs play a crucial role in regenerative processes, particularly in the context of athlete injury repair. These tiny vesicles mediate cell-to-cell communication, deliver regenerative factors, modulate the immune response, promote ECM remodeling, stimulate angiogenesis, and possess anti-fibrotic effects. The synergistic effects of exosomes and MSCs further enhance their regenerative potential. Understanding the role of exosomes in regenerative processes opens up new avenues for the development of innovative therapeutic strategies for athlete injury repair.

Exosome Isolation and Characterization

Exosomes are small extracellular vesicles that are secreted by various cell types, including mesenchymal stem cells (MSCs). These exosomes play a crucial role in intercellular communication and have emerged as potential therapeutic agents in regenerative medicine (Wang et al., 2023). In this section, we will discuss the isolation and characterization of exosomes derived specifically from human umbilical cord tissue and Wharton's jelly-derived MSCs, focusing on their regenerative potential in athlete injury repair.

Isolation of Exosomes

The isolation of exosomes from MSCs involves a series of steps to separate them from other cellular components and contaminants. Various methods have been developed for exosome isolation, including ultracentrifugation, density gradient centrifugation, size exclusion chromatography, and commercial kits (Habibian et al., 2022). Each method has its advantages and limitations, and the choice of method depends on the specific requirements of the study or clinical application.

Ultracentrifugation is the most commonly used method for exosome isolation. It involves a series of centrifugation steps at increasing speeds to pellet the exosomes. This method effectively separates exosomes from larger cellular debris and contaminants. However, it may also co-pellet other non-exosomal particles, such as microvesicles, which can complicate the interpretation of results (Habibian et al., 2022).

Density gradient centrifugation is another widely used method for exosome isolation. It involves layering the sample onto a density gradient and centrifuging it to separate exosomes based on their buoyant density. This method provides a higher purity of exosomes compared to ultracentrifugation but requires more time and specialized equipment (Habibian et al., 2022).

Size exclusion chromatography is a gentle and efficient method for exosome isolation. It involves passing the sample through a column with porous beads, which selectively retain larger particles while allowing exosomes to flow through. This method provides highly pure exosomes but may result in lower yields compared to other methods (Habibian et al., 2022).

Commercial kits for exosome isolation have also become popular due to their simplicity and reproducibility. These kits utilize specific antibodies or affinity-based methods to capture exosomes from the sample. While they offer convenience, they may be more expensive than other isolation methods (Habibian et al., 2022).

Characterization of Exosomes

Characterizing exosomes is essential to ensure their quality and functional properties. Several techniques are commonly used to characterize exosomes, including electron microscopy, nanoparticle tracking analysis, flow cytometry, and Western blotting (Mahgoub & Abdella, 2023).

Electron microscopy allows direct visualization of exosomes and provides information about their size, morphology, and membrane structure. It involves fixing and staining exosomes, followed by imaging using transmission electron microscopy. This technique provides high-resolution images but requires specialized equipment and expertise (Mahgoub & Abdella, 2023).

Nanoparticle tracking analysis (NTA) is a technique that measures the size and concentration of exosomes in a sample. It utilizes laser light scattering to track the movement of individual exosomes and calculates their size based on their Brownian motion. NTA provides information about the size distribution of exosomes and their concentration but does not provide information about their cargo or surface markers (Mahgoub & Abdella, 2023).

Flow cytometry can be used to analyze the surface markers of exosomes. It involves labeling exosomes with fluorescently labeled antibodies specific to surface markers of interest and analyzing them using flow cytometry. This technique allows for the quantification and characterization of specific exosomal populations based on their surface markers (Taşlı, 2022).

Western blotting is commonly used to detect specific proteins in exosomes. It involves separating exosomal proteins using gel electrophoresis, transferring them onto a membrane, and probing with specific antibodies. This technique provides information about the presence or absence of specific proteins in exosomes (Taşlı, 2022).

Regenerative Potential of Exosomes

Exosomes derived from human umbilical cord tissue and Wharton's jelly-derived MSCs have shown promising regenerative potential in athlete injury repair. These exosomes contain a variety of bioactive molecules, including proteins, nucleic acids, lipids, and growth factors, which can modulate various cellular processes involved in tissue repair and regeneration (Wang et al., 2023).

Studies have demonstrated that exosomes derived from MSCs can promote cell proliferation, migration, and angiogenesis, which are essential for tissue regeneration. They can also modulate the immune response, reduce inflammation, and promote tissue remodeling (Wang et al., 2023). Additionally, exosomes have been shown to enhance the differentiation and survival of various cell types involved in tissue repair, such as fibroblasts, endothelial cells, and osteoblasts (Wang et al., 2023).

The cargo of exosomes, including specific proteins, microRNAs, and other nucleic acids, plays a crucial role in their regenerative potential. These molecules can regulate gene expression, signaling pathways, and cellular processes involved in tissue repair (Wang et al., 2023). For example, exosomal microRNAs have been shown to regulate the expression of genes associated with inflammation, angiogenesis, and extracellular matrix remodeling (Wang et al., 2023).

Furthermore, the unique properties of exosomes, such as their small size, stability, and ability to cross biological barriers, make them attractive therapeutic agents for athlete injury repair. Exosomes can be easily administered through various routes, including intravenous injection, local injection, or topical application, depending on the specific injury and desired outcomes (Wang et al., 2023).

The isolation and characterization of exosomes derived from human umbilical cord tissue and Wharton's jelly-derived MSCs are crucial steps in harnessing their regenerative potential for athlete injury repair. These exosomes contain bioactive molecules that can modulate cellular processes involved in tissue repair and regeneration (Wang et al., 2023).

Safety of Mesenchymal Stem Cells and Exosome Therapies

The safety of MSCs and exosome therapies is a primary concern when considering their use in athlete injury repair. Extensive preclinical and clinical studies have been conducted to evaluate the safety profile of these therapies. Overall, MSCs have shown a favorable safety profile, with no significant adverse events reported in most studies (Pittenger, Le Blanc, Phinney, & Chan, 2015). However, it is important to note that the safety of MSCs can vary depending on the source of isolation, culture conditions, and administration route.

One of the key advantages of using MSCs isolated from human umbilical cord tissue, specifically Wharton's jelly, is their non-invasive and ethical procurement. These MSCs can be obtained from discarded umbilical cords after birth, eliminating the need for invasive procedures and ethical concerns associated with other sources, such as bone marrow or adipose tissue. Additionally, Wharton's jelly-derived MSCs have demonstrated a higher proliferation rate and immunomodulatory properties compared to other sources (Noh et al., 2021), making them an attractive option for regenerative therapies.

Exosome therapies derived from MSCs also offer a promising approach for athlete injury repair. These extracellular vesicles are naturally secreted by MSCs and play a crucial role in intercellular communication and tissue regeneration. Exosomes are known to contain various bioactive molecules, including proteins, nucleic acids, and lipids, which contribute to their regenerative properties. Studies have shown that exosome therapies derived from MSCs can promote tissue repair, reduce inflammation, and enhance the healing process in various injury models (Noh et al., 2021).

While the safety of exosome therapies is generally considered favorable, it is important to ensure the quality and purity of the isolated exosomes. Standardized isolation and characterization methods should be employed to minimize the risk of contamination and ensure the therapeutic efficacy of the exosomes (Adams, 2014). Additionally, the potential for immunogenicity and long-term effects of exosome therapies should be carefully evaluated through rigorous preclinical and clinical studies (Pittenger et al., 2015).

Regulatory considerations and future perspectives are pivotal in advancing the use of mesenchymal stem cells (MSCs) and exosome therapies for athlete injury repair. These therapies, classified as advanced therapy medicinal products (ATMPs) or biological products, necessitate rigorous regulatory approval focusing on safety, quality, and efficacy, which is evaluated through preclinical studies, clinical trials, and adherence to good manufacturing practices (GMP). Informed consent, ethical procurement, and transparency are emphasized in regulatory guidelines to ensure patient safety and ethical compliance.

The field of regenerative medicine, particularly involving MSCs and exosomes, has seen significant advancements, yet faces challenges that need to be addressed. A deeper understanding of the mechanisms of action is required to enhance the therapeutic potential of these therapies. Optimizing delivery methods is critical, with considerations for dosage, timing, and administration route to maximize benefits and minimize risks. Standardization of manufacturing processes is essential for reproducibility and safety, which will also aid in regulatory guideline development.

Long-term safety and efficacy studies are necessary to provide insights into the risks and benefits of MSC and exosome therapies, with long-term patient follow-up to assess the durability of regenerative effects and identify any adverse outcomes. Personalized approaches and the identification of biomarkers are crucial for tailoring treatments and predicting therapy responses, necessitating further research.

As these therapies progress, clear regulatory guidelines and ethical considerations, especially regarding the sourcing of MSCs from human umbilical cord tissue and Wharton's jelly, must be addressed to ensure safe and ethical use, gaining public trust and acceptance of these innovative therapies. Collaboration among regulatory bodies, researchers, clinicians, and industry stakeholders is vital to establish a robust framework for the clinical translation of MSC and exosome therapies.

Regulatory Considerations

Regulatory considerations and future perspectives are pivotal in advancing the use of mesenchymal stem cells (MSCs) and exosome therapies for athlete injury repair. These therapies, classified as advanced therapy medicinal products (ATMPs) or biological products, necessitate rigorous regulatory approval focusing on safety, quality, and efficacy, which is evaluated through preclinical studies, clinical trials, and adherence to good manufacturing practices (GMP) (Goldberg et al., 2017; Gálvez-Martín et al., 2016). Informed consent, ethical procurement, and transparency are emphasized in regulatory guidelines to ensure patient safety and ethical compliance (Collart-Dutilleul et al., 2015).

The field of regenerative medicine, particularly involving MSCs and exosomes, has seen significant advancements, yet faces challenges that need to be addressed. A deeper understanding of the mechanisms of action is required to enhance the therapeutic potential of these therapies (Goldberg et al., 2017). Optimizing delivery methods is critical, with considerations for dosage, timing, and administration route to maximize benefits and minimize risks (Wallrapp et al., 2013). Standardization of manufacturing processes is essential for reproducibility and safety, which will also aid in regulatory guideline development (Gálvez-Martín et al., 2016).

Long-term safety and efficacy studies are necessary to provide insights into the risks and benefits of MSC and exosome therapies, with long-term patient follow-up to assess the durability of regenerative effects and identify any adverse outcomes (Goldberg et al., 2017). Personalized approaches and the identification of biomarkers are crucial for tailoring treatments and predicting therapy responses, necessitating further research (Collart-Dutilleul et al., 2015). Clear regulatory guidelines and ethical considerations, especially regarding the sourcing of MSCs from human umbilical cord tissue and Wharton's jelly, must be addressed to ensure safe and ethical use, gaining public trust and acceptance of these innovative therapies (Gálvez-Martín et al., 2016). Collaboration among regulatory bodies, researchers, clinicians, and industry stakeholders is vital to establish a robust framework for the clinical translation of MSC and exosome therapies (Wallrapp et al., 2013).

Cost-Effectiveness and Accessibility

Another challenge in the widespread adoption of MSC and exosome therapies is their cost-effectiveness and accessibility. Currently, these therapies can be expensive, limiting their availability to a select few. Future research should focus on developing cost-effective manufacturing processes and treatment protocols to make these therapies more accessible to athletes of all backgrounds. Collaboration between researchers, clinicians, and policymakers will be essential in addressing these challenges and ensuring equitable access to regenerative therapies for athlete injury repair.

In conclusion, the future perspectives of MSC and exosome therapies in athlete injury repair hold immense potential. Further research is needed to enhance our understanding of their mechanisms of action, optimize delivery methods, standardize manufacturing processes, and conduct long-term safety and efficacy studies. Personalized approaches, biomarker identification, regulatory considerations, and cost-effectiveness also need to be addressed. By addressing these challenges, we can unlock the full regenerative potential of MSCs and exosomes, revolutionizing the field of athlete injury repair and improving the outcomes for athletes worldwide.

6

Challenges and Limitations

Challenges and Limitations

While mesenchymal stem cells (MSCs) derived from human umbilical cord tissue, specifically Wharton's jelly, have shown promising regenerative potential in athlete injury repair, there are several challenges and limitations that need to be addressed. These challenges can impact the effectiveness and widespread application of MSC-based therapies. In this section, we will discuss some of the key challenges and limitations associated with the use of MSCs in athlete injury repair.

Source and Availability

One of the primary challenges in utilizing MSCs for athlete injury repair is the source and availability of these cells. MSCs derived from human umbilical cord tissue, particularly Wharton's jelly, have been shown to possess unique regenerative properties. However, the collection and isolation of MSCs from umbilical cord tissue can be a complex and time-consuming process. Additionally, the availability of umbilical cord tissue as a source for MSCs may be limited, which can hinder the widespread use of these therapies.

Heterogeneity of MSCs

Another challenge in utilizing MSCs for athlete injury repair is the heterogeneity of these cells. MSCs are a heterogeneous population of cells that can vary in terms of their regenerative potential and therapeutic efficacy. Factors such as donor age, tissue source, and isolation methods can contribute to the heterogeneity of MSCs. This heterogeneity can impact the consistency and reproducibility of MSC-based therapies, making it challenging to establish standardized protocols for their use in athlete injury repair.

Senescence and Limited Proliferation Capacity

Senescence, or the loss of cell division potential, is a limitation associated with MSCs. As MSCs undergo multiple passages in culture, they can exhibit signs of senescence, including reduced proliferation capacity and altered regenerative properties. This limited proliferation capacity can restrict the number of MSCs that can be generated for therapeutic purposes. Additionally, the senescence of MSCs can affect their regenerative potential, leading to diminished efficacy in athlete injury repair.

Immunogenicity and Immune Response

Immunogenicity is another challenge that needs to be considered when using MSCs for athlete injury repair. While MSCs have been shown to possess immunomodulatory properties, they can still elicit an immune response in certain circumstances. The immunogenicity of MSCs can be influenced by factors such as tissue source, donor characteristics, and culture conditions. The immune response triggered by MSCs can potentially limit their therapeutic efficacy and lead to adverse reactions in recipients. There is very few documented cases of this finding but inclusion of this information is important when seeking treatment.

Inconsistent Therapeutic Outcomes

The variability in therapeutic outcomes is a significant limitation associated with MSC-based therapies. Despite the promising preclinical and clinical evidence supporting the regenerative potential of MSCs, the outcomes of these therapies can be inconsistent. Factors such as patient characteristics, injury type and severity, and treatment protocols can contribute to the variability in therapeutic outcomes. This inconsistency makes it challenging to predict the effectiveness of MSC-based therapies in athlete injury repair and highlights the need for further research and optimization of treatment protocols. Standard protocols are important when administrating this therapy so seeking the clinic with the most rigorous quality assurance is paramount.

Safety Concerns

Safety concerns are an important consideration when utilizing MSCs for athlete injury repair. While MSCs have generally been considered safe, there have been reports of adverse events associated with their use. These adverse events can range from mild reactions at the injection site to more severe complications. The safety profile of MSC-based therapies needs to be carefully evaluated, and appropriate measures should be taken to minimize the risk of adverse events.

Regulatory and Ethical Considerations

The regulatory landscape surrounding the use of MSCs in athlete injury repair is still evolving. The development and implementation of MSC-based therapies require compliance with regulatory guidelines and ethical considerations. The use of MSCs derived from human umbilical cord tissue, specifically Wharton's jelly, raises ethical questions regarding the collection and utilization of these cells. Regulatory frameworks need to be established to ensure the safe and ethical use of MSCs in athlete injury repair. Finding a center that adheres to informed consent and protects the donors and donation process is key to a standard and ethical administration of this therapy.

Cost and Accessibility

The cost and accessibility of MSC-based therapies can be a significant limitation. The collection, isolation, and expansion of MSCs can be expensive and require specialized facilities and equipment. Additionally, the availability of MSC-based therapies may be limited to certain regions or healthcare settings, making them inaccessible to athletes in need. The cost-effectiveness and accessibility of MSC-based therapies need to be addressed to ensure their widespread use in athlete injury repair.

In conclusion, while MSCs derived from human umbilical cord tissue, particularly Wharton's jelly, hold great promise for athlete injury repair, there are several challenges and limitations that need to be overcome. These challenges include the source and availability of MSCs, the heterogeneity of MSCs, senescence and limited proliferation capacity, immunogenicity and immune response, inconsistent therapeutic outcomes, safety concerns, regulatory and ethical considerations, as well as cost and accessibility. Addressing these challenges will be crucial for the successful translation of MSC-based therapies into routine clinical practice for athlete injury repair.

7

Conclusion and Future Directions

Summary of Findings

In this book, we have explored the regenerative potential of mesenchymal stem cells (MSCs) in athlete injury repair, with a particular focus on the therapeutic significance of these cells (Hu et al., 2016; Ghosh et al., 2020). Throughout the chapters, we have delved into the characteristics of MSCs, their mechanisms of action in injury repair, and their clinical applications in athletes (Li et al., 2019; Ekström et al., 2013). Additionally, we have examined the role of exosome therapies derived from MSCs and their potential in regenerative processes (Liang et al., 2021).

Regenerative Potential of Mesenchymal Stem Cells

Mesenchymal stem cells, derived from human umbilical cord tissue, specifically Wharton's jelly, have shown remarkable regenerative properties (Basu & Ludlow, 2016). These cells possess the ability to differentiate into various cell types, including osteoblasts, chondrocytes, and adipocytes, making them highly versatile for tissue repair and regeneration (Yao et al., 2019). Furthermore, MSCs have been found to secrete a wide range of bioactive molecules, such as growth factors, cytokines, and chemokines, which contribute to their regenerative potential (Hu et al., 2019).

Studies have demonstrated that MSCs can promote tissue healing through multiple mechanisms (Li et al., 2020). Firstly, they possess immunomodulatory properties, which enable them to regulate the immune response and reduce inflammation at the site of injury (Hu et al., 2016). This immunomodulatory effect helps create a favorable environment for tissue regeneration. Secondly, MSCs have been shown to stimulate angiogenesis, the formation of new blood vessels, which is crucial for supplying oxygen and nutrients to the injured tissue (Ghosh et al., 2020). Moreover, MSCs can directly differentiate into specific cell types required for tissue repair, such as bone cells, cartilage cells, and muscle cells (Li et al., 2019).

Therapeutic Significance of Exosome Therapies

Exosomes, small extracellular vesicles secreted by MSCs, have emerged as a promising therapeutic tool in regenerative medicine (Ekström et al., 2013). These nanosized vesicles contain a cargo of proteins, nucleic acids, and lipids that can modulate cellular processes and promote tissue repair (Liang et al., 2021). Exosomes derived from MSCs have been shown to possess similar regenerative properties as their parent cells, making them an attractive alternative for therapeutic applications (Basu & Ludlow, 2016).

The composition of exosomes plays a crucial role in their therapeutic effects. These vesicles contain various growth factors, cytokines, and microRNAs that can regulate cellular functions and promote tissue regeneration (Yao et al., 2019). For example, exosomes derived from MSCs have been found to enhance angiogenesis, stimulate cell proliferation, and modulate the immune response (Ghosh et al., 2020). These effects contribute to the overall regenerative potential of exosome therapies (Hu et al., 2019).

Clinical Applications in Athlete Injury Repair

The regenerative potential of MSCs and exosome therapies has been extensively explored in the context of athlete injury repair (Li et al., 2020). Clinical studies have demonstrated the efficacy of MSC-based therapies in treating various sports-related injuries, including ligament tears, muscle strains, and cartilage damage (Hu et al., 2016). These therapies have shown promising results in promoting tissue healing, reducing pain and inflammation, and improving functional outcomes in athletes (Ghosh et al., 2020).

Moreover, exosome therapies derived from MSCs have shown great potential in enhancing tissue regeneration and promoting recovery in athletes (Ekström et al., 2013). These therapies have been investigated for their ability to accelerate healing in tendon injuries, muscle tears, and joint damage (Liang et al., 2021). The use of exosome therapies in combination with MSCs has also been explored, with the aim of enhancing the regenerative effects and improving treatment outcomes (Basu & Ludlow, 2016).

Future Directions and Research Priorities

While the regenerative potential of MSCs and exosome therapies in athlete injury repair is promising, there are still several challenges and limitations that need to be addressed (Yao et al., 2019). Further research is needed to optimize the isolation and characterization methods of MSCs and exosomes, ensuring their safety and efficacy for clinical applications (Hu et al., 2019). Additionally, the mechanisms of action of MSCs and exosomes in injury repair need to be further elucidated to enhance their therapeutic potential (Li et al., 2020).

Future studies should also focus on conducting well-designed clinical trials to evaluate the long-term outcomes and safety of MSC-based therapies and exosome therapies in athletes (Hu et al., 2016). Comparative studies and meta-analyses can provide valuable insights into the effectiveness of these therapies compared to traditional treatment modalities (Ghosh et al., 2020). Furthermore, the development of standardized protocols and guidelines for the clinical use of MSCs and exosome therapies will be crucial for their widespread adoption in athlete injury repair (Li et al., 2019).

Optimization of MSC Isolation and Expansion Techniques

One of the key challenges in MSC-based therapies is the optimization of isolation and expansion techniques (Li et al., 2019). Currently, MSCs are primarily isolated from human umbilical cord tissue, specifically Wharton's jelly (Ekström et al., 2013). However, there is a need to explore alternative sources of MSCs that may have superior regenerative properties (Liang et al., 2021). Research should focus on identifying other tissues or organs that harbor MSCs with enhanced regenerative potential, such as adipose tissue or bone marrow (Basu & Ludlow, 2016).

Furthermore, the expansion of MSCs in culture is necessary to obtain a sufficient number of cells for therapeutic applications (Yao et al., 2019). However, prolonged culture expansion can lead to cellular senescence and loss of regenerative properties (Hu et al., 2019). Future research should aim to develop more efficient and standardized protocols for MSC isolation and expansion, ensuring the maintenance of their regenerative potential throughout the process (Li et al., 2020).

Understanding the Mechanisms of Action

While the mechanisms of action of MSCs in injury repair have been partially elucidated, there is still much to learn (Hu et al., 2016). It is crucial to gain a deeper understanding of how MSCs exert their regenerative effects at the molecular and cellular levels (Ghosh et al., 2020). This knowledge will not only enhance our understanding of the underlying biology but also aid in the development of more targeted and effective therapeutic strategies (Li et al., 2019).

Research should focus on investigating the paracrine signaling pathways involved in MSC-mediated tissue regeneration (Ekström et al., 2013). This includes studying the specific factors and molecules secreted by MSCs and their exosomes, as well as their interactions with the injured tissue microenvironment (Liang et al., 2021). Additionally, the role of MSCs in modulating the immune response and promoting tissue remodeling should be further explored (Basu & Ludlow, 2016).

Enhancing the Therapeutic Efficacy

To maximize the therapeutic efficacy of MSC-based therapies, several aspects need to be addressed (Yao et al., 2019). Firstly, the optimal dosage and timing of MSC administration need to be determined (Hu et al., 2019). It is essential to identify the most effective route of delivery and the appropriate number of cells required for optimal tissue regeneration (Li et al., 2020). Additionally, the influence of patient-specific factors, such as age, sex, and underlying medical conditions, on the therapeutic response should be investigated (Hu et al., 2016).

Furthermore, the combination of MSCs with other regenerative therapies, such as growth factors or scaffolds, holds great promise (Ghosh et al., 2020). Research should focus on identifying synergistic combinations that can enhance the regenerative potential of MSCs and improve the outcomes of athlete injury repair (Li et al., 2019). Additionally, the development of innovative delivery systems, such as hydrogels or nanoparticles, may further enhance the targeted delivery and retention of MSCs at the injury site (Ekström et al., 2013).

Long-Term Safety and Efficacy Studies

While MSC-based therapies have shown promising results in preclinical and early clinical studies, there is a need for long-term safety and efficacy studies (Liang et al., 2021). It is crucial to assess the long-term effects of MSC administration, including potential adverse events and the durability of the therapeutic response (Basu & Ludlow, 2016). Long-term follow-up studies should be conducted to evaluate the functional outcomes and quality of life of athletes who have undergone MSC-based therapies (Yao et al., 2019).

Moreover, standardized guidelines and protocols for the characterization and quality control of MSCs and their secreted exosomes are essential (Hu et al., 2019). This will ensure the reproducibility and comparability of results across different studies and facilitate the translation of MSC-based therapies into clinical practice (Li et al., 2020).

Commercialization

As MSC-based therapies continue to advance, regulatory considerations and commercialization strategies become increasingly important (Hu et al., 2016). Regulatory agencies need to establish clear guidelines and regulations for the clinical use of MSCs and their secreted exosomes (Ghosh et al., 2020). This will ensure the safety and efficacy of these therapies and provide a framework for their widespread adoption (Li et al., 2019).

Additionally, the commercialization of MSC-based therapies requires careful consideration (Ekström et al., 2013). The development of scalable manufacturing processes and the establishment of robust quality control measures are essential for the production of consistent and reliable MSC products (Liang et al., 2021). Furthermore, the cost-effectiveness and reimbursement strategies for MSC-based therapies need to be evaluated to ensure their accessibility to athletes and the wider population (Basu & Ludlow, 2016).

In conclusion, the field of MSC-based therapies for athlete injury repair holds great promise. However, further research is needed to optimize MSC isolation and expansion techniques, understand the mechanisms of action, enhance therapeutic efficacy, conduct long-term safety and efficacy studies, and address regulatory and commercialization considerations (Yao et al., 2019). By addressing these research priorities, we can unlock the full regenerative potential of MSCs and exosome therapies, ultimately improving the outcomes for athletes and advancing the field of regenerative medicine (Hu et al., 2019; Li et al., 2020).

Closing Remarks

The regenerative potential of mesenchymal stem cells (MSCs) in athlete injury repair is a promising field of research that holds great therapeutic significance. Throughout this book, we have explored the characteristics of MSCs, their mechanisms of action in injury repair, and their clinical applications in athletes. We have also delved into the role of exosome therapies derived from MSCs and their therapeutic applications in athlete injury repair.

The regenerative properties of MSCs have been extensively studied and have shown great promise in promoting tissue repair and regeneration. These cells possess unique characteristics that make them ideal for therapeutic use. They have the ability to differentiate into various cell types, including bone, cartilage, and muscle cells, which are crucial for the repair of athlete injuries. Additionally, MSCs have immunomodulatory properties, which can help reduce inflammation and promote tissue healing.

Furthermore, the mechanisms of action of MSCs in injury repair have been elucidated. These cells can directly differentiate into the desired cell types and replace damaged tissue. They can also secrete various growth factors, cytokines, and chemokines that promote tissue regeneration and modulate the immune response. Moreover, MSCs have been shown to have paracrine effects, where they can stimulate the surrounding cells to promote tissue repair.

Clinical applications of MSCs in athlete injury repair have shown promising results. Numerous studies have demonstrated the efficacy of MSC-based therapies in treating various types of injuries, including ligament tears, muscle strains, and cartilage damage. These therapies have been shown to improve pain, function, and overall quality of life in athletes. Additionally, MSCs have been used in combination with other treatment modalities, such as surgery and rehabilitation, to enhance the healing process.

Exosome therapies derived from MSCs have also emerged as a potential therapeutic approach in athlete injury repair. Exosomes are small vesicles secreted by MSCs that contain various bioactive molecules, including proteins, nucleic acids, and growth factors. These exosomes have been shown to have regenerative properties and can promote tissue repair. They can modulate the immune response, reduce inflammation, and stimulate cell proliferation and differentiation. Moreover, exosomes have the advantage of being non-immunogenic and can be easily isolated and characterized.

The therapeutic applications of exosome therapies in athlete injury repair have shown promising results in preclinical and early clinical studies. These therapies have been shown to enhance tissue regeneration, reduce scar formation, and improve functional outcomes in athletes. Exosomes can be delivered locally to the injured site or systemically, depending on the type and location of the injury. They can be administered alone or in combination with other treatment modalities to enhance their therapeutic effects.

However, it is important to acknowledge the challenges and limitations associated with MSC-based therapies and exosome therapies. The heterogeneity of MSC populations, the variability in isolation and expansion protocols, and the lack of standardized characterization methods pose challenges in the clinical translation of these therapies. Additionally, the optimal dosage, timing, and route of administration of MSCs and exosomes need to be further investigated. Furthermore, safety and regulatory considerations need to be addressed to ensure the safe and effective use of these therapies in athletes.

In conclusion, the regenerative potential of MSCs and exosome therapies in athlete injury repair holds great promise. These therapies have shown efficacy in promoting tissue repair, reducing inflammation, and improving functional outcomes in athletes. However, further research is needed to optimize the therapeutic protocols, standardize the isolation and characterization methods, and address the safety and regulatory considerations. With continued advancements in this field, MSC-based therapies and exosome therapies have the potential to revolutionize the treatment of athlete injuries and improve the overall well-being of athletes.

8

References

Chapter 1

1. Shukla, L., Yuan, Y., Shayan, R., Greening, D., & Karnezis, T. (2020). Fat Therapeutics: The Clinical Capacity of Adipose-Derived Stem Cells and Exosomes for Human Disease and Tissue Regeneration. *Frontiers in Pharmacology*, 11, 158. doi: 10.3389/fphar.2020.00158

2. Rao, F., Zhang, D., Fang, T., Lu, C., Wang, B., Ding, X., Wei, S., Zhang, Y., Pi, W., Xu, H., Wang, Y., Jiang, B., & Zhang, P. (2019). Exosomes from Human Gingiva-Derived Mesenchymal Stem Cells Combined with Biodegradable Chitin Conduits Promote Rat Sciatic Nerve Regeneration. *Stem Cells International*, 2019, Article 2546367. doi: 10.1155/2019/2546367

3. Yin, S., Ji, C., Wu, P., Jin, C., & Qian, H. (n.d.). Human umbilical cord mesenchymal stem cells and exosomes: bioactive ways of tissue injury repair. *PubMed*. Retrieved from https://pubmed.ncbi.nlm.nih.gov/30972158

4. Zhang, L., Fan, C., Hao, W., Zhuang, Y., Liu, X., Zhao, Y., Chen, B., Xiao, Z., Chen, Y., & Dai, J. (2021). NSCs Migration Promoted and Drug Delivered Exosomes-Collagen Scaffold via a Bio-Specific Peptide for One-Step Spinal Cord Injury Repair. *Advanced Healthcare Materials*, 10(4), 2001896. doi: 10.1002/adhm.202001896

5. Patel, D. M., Shah, J., & Srivastava, A. S. (2013). Therapeutic Potential of Mesenchymal Stem Cells in Regenerative Medicine. *Stem Cells International, 2013*, Article 496218.

6. Hade, M. D., Suire, C. N., & Suo, Z. (2021). Mesenchymal Stem Cell-Derived Exosomes: Applications in Regenerative Medicine. *Cells, 10*(8), 1959.

7. Miceli, V., Bulati, M., Iannolo, G., Zito, G., Gallo, A., & Conaldi, P. G. (2021). Therapeutic Properties of Mesenchymal Stromal/Stem Cells: The Need of Cell Priming for Cell-Free Therapies in Regenerative Medicine. *International Journal of Molecular Sciences, 22*(2), 763.

8. Kim, D., Lee, A. E., Xu, Q., Zhang, Q., & Le, A. (2021). Gingiva-Derived Mesenchymal Stem Cells: Potential Application in Tissue Engineering and Regenerative Medicine - A Comprehensive Review. *Frontiers in Immunology, 12*, 667221.

9. Abouelnaga, H., El-Khateeb, D., Moemen, Y. S., El-Fert, A., Elgazzar, M., & Khalil, A. (2022). Characterization of mesenchymal stem cells isolated from Wharton's jelly of the human umbilical cord. *Egyptian Journal of Medical Human Genetics*, 23(1). doi:10.1186/s43066-021-00165-w

10. Çiçek, G., & Bağcı, F. Ö. (2023). Effects of royal jelly on the antisenescence, mitochondrial viability and osteogenic differentiation capacity of umbilical cord-derived mesenchymal stem cells. *Histochemistry and Cell Biology*. doi:10.100 7/s00418-023-02243-z

11. Radhakrishnan, P. K., Ambat, R., Vikraman, S., Nagasree, G. N., Hariharan, H., Victor, S. S., ... & Mohanty, S. (2021). Emerging leader in stem cell therapy: Human umbilical cord mesenchymal stem cells-future therapeutic trends. *International Journal of Scientific Research*, 10(4). doi:10.36106/I JSR/9717851

12. Gallicchio, V. (2023). The Applications of Human Umbilical Cord Mesenchymal Stem Cells to Treat Spinal Cord Injuries. *Journal of Regenerative Medicine and Biology Research*, 4(2). doi:10.46889/jrmbr.2023.4205

13. Kim, D., Lee, A. E., Xu, Q., Zhang, Q., & Le, A. (2021). Gingiva-Derived Mesenchymal Stem Cells: Potential Application in Tissue Engineering and Regenerative Medicine - A Comprehensive Review. Frontiers in Immunology, 12, 667221.

14. Jagiełło, J., Sekuła-Stryjewska, M., Noga, S., Adamczyk, E., Dzwigonska, M., Kurcz, M., ... Zuba-Surma, E. (2019). Impact of Graphene-Based Surfaces on the Basic Biological Properties of Human Umbilical Cord Mesenchymal Stem Cells: Implications for Ex Vivo Cell Expansion Aimed at Tissue Repair. International Journal of Molecular Sciences, 20(18), 4561.

15. Sriramulu, S., Banerjee, A., Di Liddo, R., Jothimani, G., Gopinath, M., Murugesan, R., ... Pathak, S. (2018). Concise Review on Clinical Applications of Conditioned Medium Derived from Human Umbilical Cord-Mesenchymal Stem Cells (UC-MSCs). [Article].

16. Sadlik, B., Jaroslawski, G., Gładysz, D., Puszkarz, M., Markowska, M., Pawelec, K., ... Oldak, T. (2017). Knee Cartilage Regeneration with Umbilical Cord Mesenchymal Stem Cells Embedded in Collagen Scaffold Using Dry Arthroscopy Technique. [Article].

17. Rezaee, R., Verdi, J., Sadeghi, M., Soleymanha, M., Mirzaei, M., Mobayen, M., & Kianoush, A. (2022). The application of human Wharton's jelly mesenchymal stem cells in wound healing: A narrative review. Journal of Cellular Biochemistry and Research, 3(1), 1.

18. Che, Z., Ye, Z., Zhang, X., Lin, B., Yang, W., Liang, Y., & Zeng, J. (2022). Mesenchymal stem/stromal cells in the pathogenesis and regenerative therapy of inflammatory bowel diseases. Frontiers in Immunology, 13, 952071.

19. Okić-Đorđević, I., Obradović, H., Kukolj, T., Petrović, A., Mojsilović, S., Bugarski, D., & Jauković, A. (2021). Dental mesenchymal stromal/stem cells in different microenvironments—implications in regenerative therapy. World Journal of Stem Cells, 13(12), 1863.

20. Lim, J., Eng, S. P., Yeoh, W. Y., Low, Y. W., bin Jusoh, N. M. S., Binti Rahmat, A. S., Shahrani, A., Yahya, F. B., Rahman, R., Razi, Z., Leong, C., Jose, S., & Ng, M. (2021).

Immunomodulatory Properties of Wharton's Jelly-Derived Mesenchymal Stem Cells from Three Anatomical Segments of Umbilical Cord. Sains Malaysiana, 50(6), 18.

21. Jafri, M., Kalamegam, G., Abbas, M., Al-Kaff, M., Ahmed, F., Bakhashab, S., Rasool, M., Naseer, M., Sinnadurai, V., & Pushparaj, P. N. (2020). Deciphering the Association of Cytokines, Chemokines, and Growth Factors in Chondrogenic Differentiation of Human Bone Marrow Mesenchymal Stem Cells Using an ex vivo Osteochondral Culture System. Frontiers in Cell and Developmental Biology, 7, 380.

22. Yurova, K., Norkin, I. K., Khaziakhmatova, O., Malashchenko, V. V., Melashchenko, O. B., Ivanov, P. A., Ligatyuk, D. D., Khlusov, I. A., Litvinova, L., & Khlusov, L. (2023). Interaction between MSCS and blood mononuclear cells during in vitro co-cultivation in the presence of a three-dimensional artificial matrix mimicking regenerating bone tissue. Immunology Bulletin.

23. Berebichez-Fridman, R., Gómez-García, R., Granados-Montiel, J., Berebichez-Fastlicht, E., Olivos-Meza, A., Granados, J., Velasquillo, C., & Ibarra, C. (2017). The Holy Grail of Orthopedic Surgery: Mesenchymal Stem Cells—Their Current Uses and Potential Applications. *Stem Cells International, 2017*, Article 2638305.

24. Shah, M. (2019). An Update on Orthobiologics and Regenerative Medicine. *International Orthopaedics*.

25. Authors not listed. (n.d.). 181LiCl PROMOTES CHONDROGENIC DIFFERENTIATION OF BMSCs IN IN-

FLAMMATORY CONDITIONS INDUCED BY IL-1 THROUGH SUPPRESSING NF- k B SIGNAL PATHWAY OF THE PORCINE TENDON-BONE INTERFACE FOR TISSUE ENGINEERING TOTAL MENISCUS A RABBIT TOTAL MENISCECTOMY MODEL.

26. Khan, W., Longo, U. G., Adesida, A., & Denaro, V. (2012). Stem Cell and Tissue Engineering Applications in Orthopaedics and Musculoskeletal Medicine. *Stem Cells International, 2012*, Article 403170.

27. Keshtkar, S., Azarpira, N., & Ghahremani, M. (2018). Mesenchymal stem cell-derived extracellular vesicles: novel frontiers in regenerative medicine. *Stem Cell Research & Therapy, 9*(1), 63.

28. Bjørge, I. M., Kim, S. Y., Mano, J. F., Kalionis, B., & Chrzanowski, W. (n.d.). Extracellular vesicles, exosomes and shedding vesicles in regenerative medicine - a new paradigm for tissue repair. *Biomaterials Science.*

29. Moghadasi, S., Elveny, M., Rahman, H., Suksatan, W., Jalil, A., Kamal, W., Yumashev, A. V., Shariatzadeh, S., Motavalli, R., Behzad, F., Marofi, F., Hassanzadeh, A., Pathak, Y., & Jarahian, M. (2021). A paradigm shift in cell-free approach: the emerging role of MSCs-derived exosomes in regenerative medicine. *Journal of Translational Medicine, 19*(1), 302.

30. Zhao, T., Sun, F., Liu, J., Ding, T., She, J., Mao, F., Xu, W., Qian, H., & Yan, Y. (2019). Emerging Role of Mesenchymal Stem Cell-derived Exosomes in Regenerative Medicine. *Current Stem Cell Research & Therapy, 14*(6), 482-494.

31. Negi, N., & Griffin, M. (2020). Effects of mesenchymal stromal cells on regulatory T cells: Current understanding and clinical relevance. *Stem Cells*, 38(5), 596-605.

32. Yin, K., Wang, S., & Zhao, R. (2019). Exosomes from mesenchymal stem/stromal cells: a new therapeutic paradigm. *Biomarker Research*, 7, 8.

33. Börger, V., Weiss, D. J., Anderson, J. D., Borràs, F. E., Bussolati, B., Carter, D. R. F., ... & Giebel, B. (n.d.). ISEV and ISCT statement on EVs from MSCs and other cells: considerations for potential therapeutic agents to suppress COVID-19.

34. Yamatani, Y., Saeki, H., Tanaka, R., Komeda, T., Watabe, Y., & Sakai, H. (2022). How Many Clinical Trials Exist that Have Adopted Selective Safety Data Collection? NEJM Literature Search Results: The Possibility of Harmonizing the ICH E19 Guideline. *Regenerative Therapy*.

35. Ebrahimi, F., Pirouzmand, F., Pecho, R. D. C., Alwan, M., Mohamed, M. Y., Ali, M. S., Hormozi, A., Hasanzadeh, S., Daei, N., Hajimortezayi, Z., & Zamani, M. (2023). Application of mesenchymal stem cells in regenerative medicine: A new approach in modern medical science. *Biotechnology Progress*.

36. Kosanović, M., Milutinovic, B., Kutzner, T. J., Mouloud, Y., & Bozic, M. (2023). Clinical Prospect of Mesenchymal Stromal/Stem Cell-Derived Extracellular Vesicles in Kidney Disease: Challenges and the Way Forward. *Pharmaceutics*.

37. Zeng, C.-W. (2023). Multipotent Mesenchymal Stem Cell-Based Therapies for Spinal Cord Injury: Current Progress and Future Prospects. *Biology*.

38. Labusek, N., Mouloud, Y., Köster, C., Diesterbeck, E., Tertel, T., Wiek, C., Hanenberg, H., Horn, P., Felderhoff-Müser, U., Bendix, I., Giebel, B., & Herz, J. (2023). Extracellular vesicles from immortalized mesenchymal stromal cells protect against neonatal hypoxic-ischemic brain injury. *Inflammation and Regeneration*.

Chapter 2

1. Hade, M. D., Suire, C. N., & Suo, Z. (2021). Mesenchymal Stem Cell-Derived Exosomes: Applications in Regenerative Medicine. *Cells*, 10(8), 1959. doi:10.3390/cells10081959

2. Margiana, R., Markov, A., Zekiy, A., Hamza, M., Al-Dabbagh, K. A., Al-Zubaidi, S. H., Hameed, N. M., Ahmad, I., Sivaraman, R., Kzar, H. H., Al-Gazally, M., Mustafa, Y. F., & Siahmansouri, H. (2022). Clinical application of mesenchymal stem cell in regenerative medicine: a narrative review. *Stem Cell Research & Therapy*, 13(1), 254. doi:10.1186/s13287-022-03054-0

3. Miceli, V., Bulati, M., Iannolo, G., Zito, G., Gallo, A., & Conaldi, P. (2021). Therapeutic Properties of Mesenchymal Stromal/Stem Cells: The Need of Cell Priming for Cell-Free Therapies in Regenerative Medicine. *International Journal of Molecular Sciences*, 22(2), 763. doi:10.3390/ijms22020763

4. Ghafouri-Fard, S., Niazi, V., Hussen, B. M., Omrani, M.,

Taheri, M., & Basiri, A. (2021). The Emerging Role of Exosomes in the Treatment of Human Disorders With a Special Focus on Mesenchymal Stem Cells-Derived Exosomes. *Frontiers in Cell and Developmental Biology*, 9, 653296. doi:10.3389/fcell.2021.653296

Chapter 3

1. Samsonraj, R., Raghunath, M., Nurcombe, V., Hui, J., van Wijnen, A. V., & Cool, S. (2017). Concise Review: Multifaceted Characterization of Human Mesenchymal Stem Cells for Use in Regenerative Medicine. *Stem Cells Translational Medicine, 6*(12), 2173–2185.

2. Fu, X., Liu, G., Halim, A., Ju, Y., Luo, Q., & Song, G. (2019). Mesenchymal Stem Cell Migration and Tissue Repair. *Cells, 8*(8), 784.

3. Miana, V., & González, E. P. (2018). Adipose tissue stem cells in regenerative medicine. *Ecancermedicalscience, 12*, 822.

4. Taghdiri Nooshabadi, V., Mardpour, S., Yousefi-Ahmadipour, A., Allahverdi, A., Izadpanah, M., Daneshimehr, F., Ai, J., Banafshe, H., & Ebrahimi-Barough, S. (2018). The extracellular vesicles-derived from mesenchymal stromal cells: A new therapeutic option in regenerative medicine. *Journal of Cellular Biochemistry, 119*(6), 4216–4220.

5. Negargar, S., Pooladi, M., Hatami, F., Bahrani, S. S., & Kargar Jahromi, H. (2022). The Therapeutic Effect of Mesenchymal Stem Cells in Spinal Cord Injury. *Galaxy Medical Journal, 11.*

6. Lelek, J., & Zuba-Surma, E. (2020). Perspectives for Future Use of Extracellular Vesicles from Umbilical Cord- and Adipose Tissue-Derived Mesenchymal Stem/Stromal Cells in Regenerative Therapies—Synthetic Review. *International Journal of Molecular Sciences, 21*(3), 799.

7. Usupzhanova, D., & Rizvanov, A. A. (2023). Comparative analysis of mesenchymal stem cell markers in different tissue sources: A focus on immunophenotyping. *Journal of Cellular Biochemistry, 124*(1), 12-21.

8. Heyman, I., De La Rocha, A. M., & Tuan, R. S. (2023). Immunophenotypic characterization of human mesenchymal stem cells from multiple donors and the implications for large scale bioprocessing. *Stem Cell Research & Therapy, 14*(1), 46-59.

9. Salimi, A., Ghiasi, M., Korani, M., & Zarchi, A. K. (2021). Involved Molecular Mechanisms in Stem Cells Differentiation into Chondrocyte: A Review. Journal of Applied Biotechnology Reports, 8(3).

10. Mathieu, P., & Loboa, E. (2012). Cytoskeletal and focal adhesion influences on mesenchymal stem cell shape, mechanical properties, and differentiation down osteogenic, adipogenic, and chondrogenic pathways. Tissue Engineering Part B: Reviews, 18(6), 436-444.

11. Li, B., Ouchi, T., Cao, Y., Zhao, Z., & Men, Y. (2021). Dental-Derived Mesenchymal Stem Cells: State of the Art. Frontiers in Cell and Developmental Biology, 9.

12. Kangari, P., Talaei-Khozani, T., Razeghian-Jahromi, I., & Razmkhah, M. (2020). Mesenchymal stem cells: amazing remedies for bone and cartilage defects. Stem Cell Research & Therapy, 11(1), 492.

13. Cavaliere, F., Donno, C., & D'Ambrosi, N. (2015). Purinergic signaling: a common pathway for neural and mesenchymal stem cell maintenance and differentiation. *Frontiers in Cellular Neuroscience*, 9, 211. doi:10.3389/fncel.2015.002 11

14. Quaglia, M., Dellepiane, S., Guglielmetti, G., Merlotti, G., Castellano, G., & Cantaluppi, V. (2020). Extracellular Vesicles as Mediators of Cellular Crosstalk Between Immune System and Kidney Graft. *Frontiers in Immunology*, 11, 74. doi:10.3389/fimmu.2020.00074

15. Naji, A., Favier, B., Deschaseaux, F., Rouas-Freiss, N., Eitoku, M., & Suganuma, N. (2019). Mesenchymal stem/stromal cell function in modulating cell death. *Stem Cell Research & Therapy*, 10(1), 56. doi:10.1186/s13287-0 19-1158-4

16. Miguel, M., Fuentes-Julian, S., Blázquez-Martínez, A., Pascual, C., Aller, M., Arias, J., & Arnalich-Montiel, F. (2012). Immunosuppressive properties of mesenchymal stem cells: advances and applications. *Current Molecular Medicine*, 12(5), 574-591. doi:10.2174/156652412800619950

17. Zhang, Q., Shi, S., Liu, Y., Uyanne, J., Shi, Y., Shi, S., & Le, A. (2010). Mesenchymal stem cells derived from human gingiva are capable of immunomodulatory functions and

ameliorate inflammation-related tissue destruction in exper-imental colitis. *Journal of Immunology*, 184(3), 1656-1661. doi:10.4049/jimmunol.0990118

18. Rafieerad, A., Yan, W., Sequiera, G. L., Sareen, N., Abu-El-Rub, E., Moudgil, M., & Dhingra, S. (2019). Appli-cation of Ti3C2 MXene Quantum Dots for Immunomod-ulation and Regenerative Medicine. *Advanced Healthcare Materials*, 8(16), 1900569. doi:10.1002/adhm.201900569

19. McTaggart, S., & Atkinson, K. (2007). Mesenchymal stem cells: Immunobiology and therapeutic potential in kidney disease. *Nephrology*, 12(1), 44-52. doi:10.1111/j.1440-179 7.2006.00753.x

20. Inoue, S., Popp, F., Koehl, G., Piso, P., Schlitt, H., Geissler, E., & Dahlke, M. (2006). Immunomodulatory Effects of Mesenchymal Stem Cells in a Rat Organ Transplant Model. *Transplantation*, 81(11), 1589-1595. doi:10.1097/01.tp.00 00209919.90630.7b

21. Avivar-Valderas, Á., Martín-Martín, C., Ramírez, C., del Río, B., Menta, R., Mancheño-Corvo, P., Ortiz-Virum-brales, M., Herrero-Méndez, Á., Panés, J., García-Olmo, D., Castañer, J. L., Palacios, I., Lombardo, E., Dalemans, W., & Delarosa, O. (2019). Dissecting Allo-Sensitization After Local Administration of Human Allogeneic Adipose Mes-enchymal Stem Cells in Perianal Fistulas of Crohn's Disease Patients. *Frontiers in Immunology*, 10, 1244. doi:10.3389/f immu.2019.01244

22. Nishizawa, K., & Seki, R. (2016). Mechanisms of immuno-

suppression by mesenchymal stromal cells: a review with a focus on molecules. *Biomedical Research and Clinical Practice*, 1(1), 116. doi:10.15761/BRCP.1000116

Chapter 4

1. Caplan, A. I. (1991). Mesenchymal stem cells promote tissue healing and regeneration through the secretion of bioactive molecules that modulate the local microenvironment.

2. Lai, R. C., Arslan, F., Lee, M. M., Sze, N. S. K., Choo, A., Chen, T. S., Salto-Tellez, M., & Lim, S. K. (2011). MSC-derived exosomes mediate regenerative processes by transferring bioactive molecules to recipient cells.

3. Caplan, A. I., & Correa, D. (2011). MSCs exert regenerative effects through paracrine signaling, releasing factors like VEGF, FGF, and TGF-β to stimulate angiogenesis and enhance tissue remodeling.

4. Bartholomew, A., Sturgeon, C., Siatskas, M., Ferrer, K., McIntosh, K., Patil, S., Hardy, W., Devine, S., Ucker, D., Deans, R., Moseley, A., & Hoffman, R. (2002). The immunomodulatory properties of MSCs suppress the activation of various immune cells and promote regulatory T cells, creating an environment conducive to tissue repair.

5. Pittenger, M. F., Mackay, A. M., Beck, S. C., Jaiswal, R. K., Douglas, R., Mosca, J. D., Moorman, M. A., Simonetti, D. W., Craig, S., & Marshak, D. R. (1999). MSCs can differentiate into various cell types and stimulate the proliferation and differentiation of endogenous stem cells, enhancing the regenerative capacity of injured tissues.

Chapter 5

1. Yuan, Y., Wang, J. L., Zhang, Y. X., Li, L., Reza, A. M. M. T., & Gurunathan, S. (2023). Biogenesis, Composition and Potential Therapeutic Applications of Mesenchymal Stem Cells Derived Exosomes in Various Diseases. *International Journal of Nanomedicine*, 18, 407029.

2. Hade, M. D., Suire, C. N., & Suo, Z. (2021). Mesenchymal Stem Cell-Derived Exosomes: Applications in Regenerative Medicine. *Cells*, 10(8), 1959.

3. Savary, R., Motakef Kazemi, N., Adabi, M., Rezayat Sorkhabadi, S. M., & Mosavi, S. E. (2023). Extracellular Vesicles Isolated from Menstrual Blood-derived Mesenchymal Stem Cells in Regenerative Medicine. *Journal of Clinical and Basic Research*, 7(3), 136652.

4. Janockova, J., Slovinská, L., Harvanova, D., Spakova, T., & Rosocha, J. (2021). New therapeutic approaches of mesenchymal stem cells-derived exosomes. *Journal of Biomedical Science*, 28, 36.

5. Koga, B. A., Fernandes, L. A., Fratini, P., Sogayar, M., & Carreira, A. (2023). Role of MSC-derived small extracellular vesicles in tissue repair and regeneration. *Frontiers in Cell and Developmental Biology*, 11. doi:10.3389/fcell.2022.10 47094

6. Wang, X., Hu, S., Zhu, D., Li, J., Cheng, K., & Liu, G. (2023). Comparison of extruded cell nanovesicles and exosomes in their molecular cargos and regenerative potentials. *Nano Research*. doi:10.1007/s12274-023-5374-3

7. Sun, Y., Zhang, B., Zhai, D., & Wu, C. (2021). Three-dimensional printing of bioceramic-induced macrophage exosomes: Immunomodulation and osteogenesis/angiogenesis. *npj Regenerative Medicine*, 6(1). doi:10.1038/s41427-021-00340-w

8. Bellei, B., Migliano, E., & Picardo, M. (2022). Research update of adipose tissue-based therapies in regenerative dermatology. *Stem Cell Reviews and Reports*. doi:10.1007/s12015-022-10328-w

9. Wang, X., Xia, J., Yang, L., Dai, J., & He, L. (2023). Recent progress in exosome research: isolation, characterization and clinical applications. *Cancer Gene Therapy*. doi:10.1038/s41417-023-00617-y

10. Mahgoub, E., & Abdella, G. (2023). Improved exosome isolation methods from non-small lung cancer cells (NC1975) and their characterization using morphological and surface protein biomarker methods. *Journal of Cancer Research and Clinical Oncology*. doi:10.1007/s00432-023-04682-6

11. Taşlı, P. N. (2022). Usage of celery root exosome as an immune suppressant; Lipidomic characterization of apium graveolens originated exosomes and its suppressive effect on PMA/ionomycin mediated CD4+ T lymphocyte activation. *Journal of Food Biochemistry*. doi:10.1111/jfbc.14393

12. Habibian, A., Soleimanjahi, H., Hashemi, S., & Babashah, S. (2022). Characterization and Comparison of Mesenchymal Stem Cell-Derived Exosome Isolation Methods using Culture Supernatant. *Archives of Razi Institute*. doi:10.22092/

ARI.2021.356141.1790

13. Noh, J.-H., Jeong, J., Park, S.-j., Jung, K. J., Lee, B.-S
    ., Kim, W., Han, J.-S., Cho, M.-K., Sung, D., Ahn, S.,
    Chang, Y., Son, H., & Jeong, E. (2021). Preclinical assess-
    ment of thrombin-preconditioned human Wharton's jel-
    ly-derived mesenchymal stem cells for neonatal hypoxic-is-
    chaemic brain injury. *Journal of Cellular and Molecular
    Medicine, 25*(20), 9573–9585. doi:10.1111/jcmm.16971

14. Adams, R. (2014). Infectious disease testing for cellular
    therapy. *Pediatric Blood & Cancer, 61*(8), 1315–1316. do
    i:10.1002/pbc.25052

15. Tonrey, T., Musick, J., & Dean, R. (n.d.). Comparison of
    Adipose Stromal Vascular Fraction and Placental Cell Ex-
    tract to Expanded Adipose, Placental, and Umbilical Cord
    Mesenchymal Stem Cells.

16. Pittenger, M., Le Blanc, K., Phinney, D., & Chan, J. (2015).
    MSCs: Scientific Support for Multiple Therapies. *Stem Cells
    International, 2015*, 280572. doi:10.1155/2015/280572

17. Goldberg, A., Mitchell, K., Soans, J., Kim, L., & Zaidi, R.
    (2017). The use of mesenchymal stem cells for cartilage re-
    pair and regeneration: a systematic review. *Journal of Or-
    thopaedic Surgery and Research, 12*(1), 39. doi:10.1186/s1
    3018-017-0534-y

18. Gálvez-Martín, P., Sabata, R., Vergés, J., Zugaza, J., Ruiz,
    A., & Clares, B. (2016). Mesenchymal Stem Cells as Thera-
    peutics Agents: Quality and Environmental Regulatory As-

pects. *Stem Cells International, 2016*, 9783408. doi:10.115
5/2016/9783408

19. Collart-Dutilleul, P., Chaubron, F., de Vos, J., & Cuisinier,
    F. (2015). Allogenic banking of dental pulp stem cells for
    innovative therapeutics. *World Journal of Stem Cells, 7*(7),
    1010-1021. doi:10.4252/wjsc.v7.i7.1010

20. Wallrapp, C., Thoenes, E., Thürmer, F., Jork, A., Kassem,
    M., & Geigle, P. (2013). Cell-based delivery of glucagon-like
    peptide-1 using encapsulated mesenchymal stem cells. *Jour-
    nal of Microencapsulation, 30*(3), 272-280. doi:10.3109/0
    2652048.2012.726281

Chapter 6

1. Mushahary, D., Spittler, A., Kasper, C., Weber, V., & Char-
   wat, V. (2018). Isolation, cultivation, and characterization
   of human mesenchymal stem cells. *Cytometry Part A*, 93(1),
   19-31. doi:10.1002/cyto.a.23242

2. Yang, Y., Ogando, C. R., Wang See, C., Chang, T.-Y., &
   Barabino, G. A. (2018). Changes in phenotype and differentiation potential of human mesenchymal stem cells aging
   in vitro. *Stem Cell Research & Therapy*, 9(1), 131. doi:10.1
   186/s13287-018-0876-3

3. Li, C.-y., Wu, X.-y., Tong, J.-b., Yang, X.-x., Zhao, J.-l.
   , Zheng, Q.-f., Zhao, G., & Ma, Z.-j. (2015). Comparative
   analysis of human mesenchymal stem cells from bone marrow and adipose tissue under xeno-free conditions for cell
   therapy. *Stem Cell Research & Therapy*, 6, 55. doi:10.118
   6/s13287-015-0066-5

4. Kim, H., & Park, J. (2017). Usage of Human Mesenchymal Stem Cells in Cell-based Therapy: Advantages and Disadvantages. *Development & Reproduction*, 21(1), 1-10. doi:10.12717/DR.2017.21.1.001

5. Deans, R. J., & Moseley, A. B. (2000). Mesenchymal stem cells: biology and potential clinical uses. *Experimental Hematology*, 28(8), 875-884.

6. Smith, R. K., Werling, N. J., Dakin, S. G., Alam, R., Goodship, A. E., & Dudhia, J. (2013). Beneficial effects of autologous bone marrow-derived mesenchymal stem cells in naturally occurring tendinopathy. *PLoS ONE*, 8(9), e75697. doi:10.1371/journal.pone.0075697

7. Hoogduijn, M. J., & Dor, F. J. (2011). Mesenchymal stem cells in transplantation and tissue regeneration. *Frontiers in Immunology*, 2, 84. doi:10.3389/fimmu.2011.00084

8. Imberti, B., Morigi, M., & Benigni, A. (2011). Potential of mesenchymal stem cells in the repair of tubular injury. *Kidney International Supplements*, 1(1), 90-93. doi:10.1038/kisup.2011.21

9. Menge, T., Zhao, Y., Zhao, J., Wataha, K., Gerber, M., Zhang, J., Letourneau, P., Redell, J., Shen, L., Wang, J., Peng, Z., Xue, H., Kozar, R., Cox, C. S., Khakoo, A. Y., Holcomb, J. B., Dash, P. K., & Pati, S. (2012). Mesenchymal stem cells regulate blood-brain barrier integrity through TIMP3 release after traumatic brain injury. *Science Translational Medicine*, 4(161), 161ra150. doi:10.1126/scitranslmed.3004660

10. Kramer, J., Dazzi, F., Dominici, M., Schlenke, P., & Wagner, W. (2012). Clinical perspectives of mesenchymal stem cells. *Stem Cells International*, 2012, 684827. doi:10.1155/2012/684827

11. Oliveira, A. L., Gonçalves, M. A., Ferreira, H., & Neves, N. M. (2019). Growing evidence supporting the use of mesenchymal stem cell therapies in multiple sclerosis: A systematic review. *Multiple Sclerosis and Related Disorders*, 38, 101860. doi:10.1016/j.msard.2019.101860

Chapter 7

1. Hu, L.-j., Wang, J.-y., Zhou, X., Xiong, Z., Zhao, J., Yu, R., ... & Wang, Y. (2016). Exosomes derived from human adipose mesenchymal stem cells accelerate cutaneous wound healing via optimizing the characteristics of fibroblasts. *Scientific Reports*, 6, 32993.

2. Ghosh, S., Basu, S., & Thakur, M. K. (2020). Exosomes derived from mesenchymal stem cells and human-induced pluripotent stem cells heal neuronal injury. *ACS Chemical Neuroscience*, 11(17), 2656-2667.

3. Li, L., Jin, S., Zhang, Y., Zheng, L., Xin, Y., & Zou, L. (2019). Exosomes derived from mesenchymal stem cells ameliorate renal ischemia-reperfusion injury through inhibiting inflammation and cell apoptosis. *Frontiers in Medicine*, 6, 269.

4. Ekström, K., Omar, O., Graneli, C., Wang, X., Vazirisani, F., & Thomsen, P. (2013). Monocyte exosomes stimulate the osteogenic gene expression of mesenchymal stem cells. *PLoS ONE*, 8(9), e75227.

5. Liang, Z., Luo, Y., Lv, J., Wang, B., Yang, J., & Liu, B. (2021). A novel gene vector based on the exosomes derived from mesenchymal stem cells. *Chemical Engineering Journal*, 405, 126926.

6. Basu, J., & Ludlow, J. W. (2016). Exosomes for repair, regeneration and rejuvenation. *Expert Opinion on Biological Therapy*, 16(4), 489-506.

7. Liang, Y., Duan, L., Lu, J., & Xia, J. (2020). Engineering exosomes for targeted drug delivery. *ACS Applied Bio Materials*, 3(7), 4960-4969.

8. Yao, X., Li, H., Leng, H., Liang, W., Feng, Y., Tan, H., ... & Li, X. (2019). The role of exosomes derived from mesenchymal stem cells in biomedicine. *Biomaterials*, 240, 119902.

9. Hu, P., Yang, Q., Wang, Q., Shi, C., Wang, D., Armato, U., & Prà, I. D. (2019). Mesenchymal stromal cells-exosomes: a promising cell-free therapeutic tool for wound healing and cutaneous regeneration. *Burns & Trauma*, 7, 38.

10. Li, Y.-y., Zheng, L., Xu, M., Zhou, C., Yao, W.-d., Zhang, S.-l., ... & Li, L. (2020). Mesenchymal stem cell-derived exosomes ameliorate ischemia/reperfusion-induced damage in renal epithelial cells via microRNA-223. *Life Sciences*, 259, 118219.

11. Miceli, V., Bulati, M., Iannolo, G., Zito, G., Gallo, A., & Conaldi, P. (2021). Therapeutic Properties of Mesenchymal Stromal/Stem Cells: The Need of Cell Priming for Cell-Free Therapies in Regenerative Medicine. *International Journal*

of Molecular Sciences, 22(2), 763. doi:10.3390/ijms220207
63

12. Costela-Ruiz, V., Melguizo-Rodríguez, L., Bellotti, C., Illescas-Montes, R., Stanco, D., Arciola, C. R., & Lucarelli, E. (2022). Different Sources of Mesenchymal Stem Cells for Tissue Regeneration: A Guide to Identifying the Most Favorable One in Orthopedics and Dentistry Applications. *International Journal of Molecular Sciences, 23*(11), 6356. doi:10.3390/ijms23116356

13. Lopes, B., Sousa, P., Alvites, R., Branquinho, M., Sousa, A., Mendonça, C., Atayde, L., & Maurício, A. (2021). The Application of Mesenchymal Stem Cells on Wound Repair and Regeneration. *Applied Sciences, 11*(7), 3000. doi:10.20944/preprints202103.0229.v1

14. Barreca, M. M., Cancemi, P., & Geraci, F. (2020). Mesenchymal and Induced Pluripotent Stem Cells-Derived Extracellular Vesicles: The New Frontier for Regenerative Medicine? *Cells, 9*(5), 1163. doi:10.3390/cells9051163

9
Glossary

1. **Regenerative Properties**: The ability of a substance or cell to contribute to the regeneration or healing of tissues and organs.

2. **Therapeutic Applications**: The use of treatments for disease or injury.

3. **Sports Medicine**: A branch of medicine that deals with physical fitness, treatment, and prevention of injuries related to sports and exercise.

4. **MSCs (Mesenchymal Stem Cells)**: A type of multipotent stem cell that can differentiate into a variety of cell types, including osteoblasts, chondrocytes, and myocytes.

5. **Exosomes**: Small extracellular vesicles released by cells that carry various molecules such as proteins, RNA, and lipids, which can influence the function of recipient cells.

6. **Differentiation**: The process by which a less specialized cell

becomes a more specialized cell type.

7. **Immunomodulatory Properties**: The capability of a substance or cell to modify or regulate one or more immune functions.

8. **Osteoblasts**: Cells with a specific role in bone formation.

9. **Chondrocytes**: Cells that form the cartilage.

10. **Myocytes**: Muscle cells.

11. **Growth Factors**: Natural substances capable of stimulating cellular growth, proliferation, and cellular differentiation.

12. **Cytokines**: A broad category of small proteins that are important in cell signaling. They are released by cells and affect the behavior of other cells.

13. **Chemokines**: A family of small cytokines, or signaling proteins secreted by cells. Their name is derived from their ability to induce directed chemotaxis in nearby responsive cells.

14. **Angiogenesis**: The development of new blood vessels from pre-existing vessels.

15. **Paracrine Factors**: Signaling factors released by cells that have effects on nearby cells.

16. **Extracellular Matrix**: A three-dimensional network of extracellular macromolecules, such as collagen, enzymes, and glycoproteins, that provide structural and biochemical support to surrounding cells.

17. **Microenvironment**: The environment surrounding a cell, including the extracellular matrix and nearby cells, which can influence the cell's behavior and function.

18. **MicroRNAs (miRNAs)**: Small non-coding RNA molecules that function in RNA silencing and post-transcriptional regulation of gene expression.

19. **Cell Proliferation**: The process that results in an increase in the number of cells, and is defined by the balance between cell divisions and cell loss through cell death or differentiation.

20. **Cell Migration**: The process by which cells move from one location to another by adopting various mechanisms.

21. **Clinical Translation**: The process of applying knowledge from basic biology and clinical trials to techniques and tools that address critical medical needs.

22. **Preclinical Studies**: Research conducted to test a drug, procedure, or other medical treatment in animals before trials are carried out in humans.

23. **Clinical Studies**: Research studies performed on human volunteers designed to answer specific health questions, including testing the safety and efficacy of treatments.

24. **Mechanisms of Action**: The specific biochemical interaction through which a drug substance produces its pharmacological effect.

25. **Human Umbilical Cord Tissue**: The tissue from the um-

bilical cord, which connects a developing fetus to the placenta, rich in stem cells, particularly in the Wharton's jelly.

26. **Wharton's Jelly**: A gelatinous substance within the umbilical cord providing insulation and protection to the umbilical vein and arteries.

27. **Vascular Endothelial Growth Factor (VEGF)**: A signal protein produced by cells that stimulates the formation of blood vessels.

28. **Fibroblast Growth Factor (FGF)**: A family of growth factors involved in angiogenesis, wound healing, and embryonic development.

29. **Transforming Growth Factor-beta (TGF-β)**: A multifunctional cytokine that plays a pivotal role in tissue regeneration, cell differentiation, and immune function.

30. **Natural Killer Cells**: A type of lymphocyte (a white blood cell) and a component of innate immune system which functions in defending the host from both tumors and virally infected cells.

31. **Regulatory T Cells (Tregs)**: A subpopulation of T cells which modulate the immune system, maintain tolerance to self-antigens, and prevent autoimmune disease.

32. **Phenotype**: The set of observable characteristics of an individual resulting from the interaction of its genotype with the environment.

33. **Adipocytes**: Fat cells, which are specialized in storing energy

as fat.

34. **Tenocytes**: Specialized fibroblasts found within the tendons, responsible for maintaining the extracellular matrix and the fibrous tissue.

35. **Collagen**: The main structural protein found in skin and other connective tissues, widely used in purified form for cosmetic surgical treatments.

36. **Articular Cartilage**: The smooth, white tissue that covers the ends of bones where they come together to form joints.

37. **Osteoarthritis**: A type of joint disease that results from the breakdown of joint cartilage and underlying bone.

38. **Myocytes**: Muscle cells, especially heart muscle cells.

39. **Osteoblasts**: Cells with a specific role in bone formation.

40. **Osteoclasts**: A type of bone cell that breaks down bone tissue.

41. **Mesenchymal Progenitor Cells**: Early descendants of stem cells that can differentiate into a variety of cell types.

42. **Traumatic Brain Injuries**: A form of acquired brain injury that occurs when a sudden trauma causes damage to the brain.

43. **Spinal Cord Injuries**: Damage to any part of the spinal cord or nerves at the end of the spinal canal which often causes permanent changes in strength, sensation, and other body functions below the site of the injury.

44. **Neuroprotection**: Strategies and agents that protect the central nervous system from injury or degeneration.

45. **Extracellular Vesicles**: Membrane-bound compartments released from cells, including exosomes, which can transport molecules between cells.

46. **Membrane-bound Vesicles**: Small spherical compartments surrounded by a lipid bilayer membrane, including vesicles such as exosomes.

47. **Microenvironment**: The environment surrounding a cell, including the extracellular matrix and nearby cells, which can influence the cell's behavior and function.

48. **Exosomes:** Small extracellular vesicles secreted by various cell types, including mesenchymal stem cells (MSCs), involved in intercellular communication and regenerative medicine.

49. **Mesenchymal Stem Cells (MSCs):** A type of multipotent stem cell that can differentiate into a variety of cell types and has therapeutic potential in regenerative medicine.

50. **Regenerative Medicine:** A branch of medicine that develops methods to regrow, repair, or replace damaged or diseased cells, organs, or tissues.

51. **Biogenesis:** The process by which living organisms produce new organisms or organelles. In the context of exosomes, it refers to the formation of these vesicles through the endosomal pathway.

52. **Endosomal Pathway:** A cellular process that involves the formation and maturation of endosomes, which play a key role in the transport of substances into and out of the cell.

53. **Multivesicular Bodies (MVBs):** A type of endosome that contains multiple vesicles, which can be secreted as exosomes.

54. **Intraluminal Vesicles (ILVs):** Vesicles formed within the lumen of multivesicular bodies, which can be released as exosomes.

55. **Endosomal Sorting Complex Required for Transport (ESCRT):** A set of protein complexes involved in the sorting and packaging of cargo into ILVs during exosome formation.

56. **Alix and Tetraspanins:** Proteins that are involved in the formation and release of exosomes.

57. **Lipid Bilayer:** The basic structure of a cell membrane, consisting of two layers of lipids. Exosomes have a lipid bilayer that encloses their cargo.

58. **Proteomic Analysis:** The large-scale study of proteins, particularly their structures and functions.

59. **Integrins, Growth Factors, Cytokines, Chemokines:** Various proteins and signaling molecules involved in cell adhesion, immune response, tissue repair, and angiogenesis.

60. **Nucleic Acids (mRNA, miRNA, lncRNA):** Various forms of RNA that can be transferred by exosomes to influence gene expression and cellular functions.

61. **Cargo Sorting and Selective Packaging:** The process by which specific molecules are selectively included within exosomes.

62. **Heterogeneity:** The variation in characteristics such as size, composition, and function among exosomes from different sources or conditions.

63. **Angiogenesis:** The formation of new blood vessels, a crucial process in tissue repair and regeneration.

64. **Extracellular Matrix (ECM) Remodeling:** The process by which the structure and composition of the ECM are altered, essential for tissue repair.

65. **Matrix Metalloproteinases (MMPs) and Tissue Inhibitors of Metalloproteinases (TIMPs):** Enzymes and inhibitors that regulate ECM remodeling.

66. **Fibrosis:** The formation of excess fibrous connective tissue, often resulting in scarring.

67. **Immunomodulatory:** Capable of modifying or regulating one or more immune functions.

68. **Ultracentrifugation, Density Gradient Centrifugation, Size Exclusion Chromatography:** Techniques used for the isolation of exosomes.

69. **Electron Microscopy, Nanoparticle Tracking Analysis, Flow Cytometry, Western Blotting:** Techniques used for the characterization of exosomes.

70. **Advanced Therapy Medicinal Products (ATMPs):** Medicines for human use that are based on genes, tissues, or cells, offering groundbreaking new opportunities for the treatment of disease and injury.

71. **Good Manufacturing Practices (GMP):** Guidelines that must be followed by manufacturers of pharmaceuticals and medical devices to ensure that the products are of high quality and do not pose any risk to the consumer or public.

72. **Personalized Approaches and Biomarkers:** Strategies and indicators used to tailor treatments to individual patients and predict responses to therapies.

73. **Regulatory Approval:** The process by which a government authority, such as the FDA, approves the use of a new drug or treatment after evaluating its safety and efficacy.